THE POLITICS OF PANDEMICS

EVOLVING REGIME-OPPOSITION DYNAMICS IN THE MENA REGION

edited by Karim Mezran and Annalisa Perteghella

ISPI

Atlantic Council

© 2020 Ledizioni LediPublishing
Via Antonio Boselli, 10 – 20136 Milan – Italy
www.ledizioni.it
info@ledizioni.it

THE POLITICS OF PANDEMICS:
EVOLVING REGIME-OPPOSITION DYNAMICS IN THE MENA REGION

Edited by Karim Mezran and Annalisa Perteghella
First edition: December 2020

Print ISBN   9788855263801
ePub ISBN   9788855263818
Pdf ISBN   9788855263825
DOI   10.14672/55263801

ISPI. Via Clerici, 5
20121, Milan
www.ispionline.it

Catalogue and reprints information: www.ledizioni.it

Atlantic Council

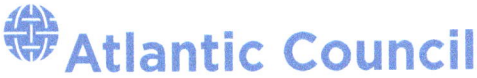

The Atlantic Council is a nonpartisan organization that promotes constructive US leadership and engagement in international affairs based on the central role of the Atlantic community in meeting today's global challenges.

Table of Contents

Preface

After the first official cases reported in Iran in late February 2020, the Covid-19 pandemic has rapidly spread to all countries in the Middle East and North Africa (MENA) region, affecting all areas of life and becoming one of the most significant factors affecting regional developments. The outbreak, whose devastating effects cannot yet be fully appreciated, could not have come at a worse time, as many countries remain engulfed in vicious internal conflicts, or must cope with structural socio-economic distress and popular dissent. In many respects, such a context and many of its problems resemble those that formed the backdrop of the Arab spring in 2011.

Ten years after those momentous events, much ink has been spilled about the drivers, dynamics and consequences of the uprisings, as well as their lasting legacy. Attention has been devoted in particular to the security and military developments that have unfolded since, either in the form of civil wars such as those in Libya, Syria, or Yemen, or in their worrisome evolutions into regionalized or internationalized conflicts, characterized by heavily entrenched zero-sum calculations. Notwithstanding the relevance of the security realm, however, some of the root causes of the Arab Springs pertain to the social and political spheres and remain to a large extent unaddressed in many countries of the region. Socio-economic inequalities, unemployment, weak governance, socio-political exclusion and ethno-religious discrimination are amongst the most relevant factors, and they all seem to converge into what could be generally defined as a "social contract".

The erosion of this social contract not only underlies the persistent occurrence of social protests and anti-governmental mobilization across the region, but it also explains the (perceived or real) widening gap between common citizens and political elites, as well as the latters' failure to meet the formers' demands. The cases of Algeria and Iraq, in particular, plainly illustrate the failure of the redistributive model of the social contract, with protesters and activists that for more than a year have been tirelessly calling for more jobs, better services, and a profound overhaul of a power system driven by corruption and cronyism. As a second wave of protests has again recently rocked parts of the Middle East and North Africa, the reaction of the authorities has been for the most part a repressive one (sometimes even leading to violence as in the case of Iraq), forestalling any significant change.

Against this backdrop, thus, the introduction of an unexpected variable such as a public health emergency due to a worldwide pandemic could potentially trigger an unprecedented reshuffle of both domestic and regional dynamics. In a nutshell, the virus has dramatically exposed the governance failures of many current administrations, as well as pre-existing vulnerabilities, exacerbating the same economic grievances that led to the recent string of popular protests in the first place. Although initially downplayed by many regional governments, the pandemic has soon made its effects felt on the economic and social spheres while pushing healthcare systems to the limit, especially in conflict-ridden or fragile countries such as Libya, Syria, and Iraq. To varying degrees, state authorities reluctantly decided to suspend economic activities, reduce trade relations, close national borders, and impose more or less severe quarantine measures to curb the spread of the disease and protect communities at risk. While some countries are faring better than others, the pandemic is expected to leave long lasting scars almost everywhere.

This report collects contributions from international experts and scholars on Middle Eastern affairs. The authors offer different perspectives on the consequences that the pandemic is having on regimes and societies in the MENA region. By focusing on six case studies that range from North African countries to the Middle East and the Gulf, this volume aims to draw a detailed and updated picture of the evolving relations between state and society, paying specific attention to the variety of regime-oppositions dynamics. Notably, this analysis takes into consideration the challenges faced by governments and rulers in their attempt to maintain a hold on increasingly unstable societies and political systems, as well as how these efforts influence their interaction with other actors in the region.

As Emadeddin Badi argues, Libya has so far been overwhelmed by the Covid-19 outbreak, with healthcare structures and medical capabilities devastated by years of war and any form of public response impeded or delayed by both military operations and the country's division into two competing governments. Here, the pandemic has not halted the war, now in a low-intensity phase, nor has it prompted any significant change in the attitudes of Libyan political elites, rather amplifying the gap with local constituencies and setting the stage for what Badi describes as a situation similar to a "*tragedy of the commons*".

In other contexts, such as in Algeria and Egpyt, the pandemic seems to have reinforced or augmented the tendence towards authoritarian rule, at least in the short term. As Yahia Mohamed Lemine Mestek recounts, Algiers and Cairo has exploited the Covid-19 emergency to enact severe – albeit temporary – social control legislations and weaken potential opponents and critics in order to cement their hold on power. In Algeria, several leaders and activists of the almost two-year-long protest movement known as *Hirak* have been imprisoned, while the government is using the pandemic to buy time and drive the country through a smooth political transition while trying to cope with a worsening economic situation. Yet, as long as the protesters' demands will be ignored or only partially recognized, buying time will only push the population to distance itself from the elite, postponing but not cancelling the need for the concrete change the people are asking for.

Turning to Egypt, Hafsa Halawa argues that for the Egyptian President Abdel Fattah Al Sisi the Covid-19 outbreak has provided a favourable context for his policies of state control. According to Halawa, Al Sisi can continue to expand the military's control over the state's institutions and the economy, while moving towards a *de facto* authoritarian system, oblivious to the fact that apparent political inactivity on the part of the opposition could actually conceal a higher degree of political awareness that may inspire anti-regime mobilization in the future.

In Baghdad, the government led by Mustafa al-Kadhimi, which was sworn in in early May, inherited from the previous administration months of violent popular protests against corruption and poor governance, tense relations with Turkey and the risk of a US-Iran confrontation on Iraqi soil. And then, the pandemic hit. As Abbas Kadhim recounts, the virus propagated and overcame an unprepared health-care system, popular mobilization receded, Iraqi streets emptied, and political elites enjoyed a temporary relief. However, most of the structural problems plaguing the country have not disappeared, and could instead worsen due to the pandemic, stoking new and stronger opposition and forcing the regime to either pursue reforms and mend fences with the political and social opposition, or continue along a path of reckless apathy.

Moving to the Arab Gulf, Gawdat Bahgat explains that these countries can count on overall solid and modern medical services. Arab Gulf countries were among the first to introduce partial or full lockdowns, together with stimulus packages aimed at sustaining domestic economies in the face of the economic slowdown and substantial financial losses caused by plunging oil prices. In fact, the combination of global supply-demand shocks and nosediving energy prices has put additional strains on even the region's wealthiest countries and may generate unprecedented tensions between governing elites and ordinary citizens.

Finally, turning to Iran, Nadereh Chamlou argues that the Iranian regime has tried to capitalize on the pandemic to tighten its rule, in spite of the catastrophic impact the virus is having in terms of human losses and economic fallout. Indeed, as of mid-November 2020, the country recorded close to 40 thousand deaths and remains the hardest-hit in the region. Besides exposing the country's structural deficiencies on many fronts, the virus has put the spotlight on the growing popular discontent towards the regime when it comes to fair justice and institutional accountability.

Overall, a more in-depth analysis of how governments have reacted to the pandemic reveals that autocrats, besides implementing emergency laws to effectively slow viral transmission, have been similarly worried about silencing those who exposed the impact that the pandemic is having on deep-seated issues affecting their own countries. This, in turn, has justified the upsurge of securitization and the deployment of repressive tools against the opposition under the guise of managing the epidemic. By means of new technologies to track citizens, extraordinary authority to impose social control measures, and emergency laws, the pandemic has also laid the foundation for future repressions. As a result, highly securitized regimes of the MENA region have seized this opportunity to keep at bay what has previously been a robust and widespread wave of discontent, and actively seek to prevent its recurrence.

Nevertheless, the pandemic has also brought to the fore the utter untenability of the social contract existing in many regional countries, exacerbating structural problems and deepening the gap between political elites and ordinary citizens. By exposing the real nature of many political regimes, the virus has also opened new spaces of dissent and forced socio-political oppositions to rethink their engagement in the face of increased pressure from the authorities, likely spreading the seeds of future mobilizations.

Frederick Kempe   *Giampiero Massolo*
President and CEO, Atlantic Council   *President, ISPI*

1. Covid-19 and Libya's Tragedy of the Commons

Emadeddin Badi

The Covid-19 pandemic has overwhelmed some of the most developed and technologically advanced healthcare systems worldwide, in addition to threatening the global economy. It has also triggered a tilt towards more autocratic policy options as even some of the most democratically leaning states have faced challenges in terms of securing the compliance of their populations to preventative social distancing measures. In the MENA region, states' pre-existing vulnerabilities in the economic, social, and political spheres have also been exacerbated. The region's governing authorities' have either failed the test of wielding tools of governance as their public health response foundered or are likely to retain and usurp the special powers they have deployed to contain the spread. Libya, a divided state that has been decaying for the past nine years, is likely to be the theater of an idiosyncratic combination of both scenarios.

Libya's healthcare system, already frail and underdeveloped during the Gaddafi era, has experienced continuous deterioration over the years that followed the revolution. The country was thus, by design, particularly vulnerable to a severe Covid-19 outbreak. Without doubt, the contemporary spread of the virus is having devastating public health implications, with health facilities across the country being already overwhelmed.[1] The

---

[1] S. Creta, "Libyan Doctors Battle On Two Dangerous Fronts: Covid-19 And

pandemic has also negatively affected the country's political economy and has exacerbated pre-existing social rifts that had already been laid bare by the civil war ignited by General Khalifa Haftar and his Libyan Arab Armed Forces (LAAF) with the launch of an offensive on Libya's capital - Tripoli - in April 2019. Amidst an already precarious situation characterized by scarcity of resources and supply shortages, Covid-19 has also brought to light institutional cracks that put populations such as migrants, refugees, and internally displaced people (IDPs) – already at the margins of service delivery – in even more vulnerable positions.

Libya's first case of Covid-19 was identified on 24 March, 2020. Though the magnitude of the spread was somewhat limited in the first two months that followed, cases have exponentially increased since July, with over 29,000 total cases being reported in September 2020 as per Libya's National Centre for Disease Control (NCDC). Of these, 460 have died and some 15,913 have recovered.[2] Yet, official statistics do not accurately reflect the real number of cases, which are likely underreported owing to limited testing capacities. Monitoring the outbreak in Libya is particularly challenging: a little under 50,000 tests have been conducted, with over half of these being in Tripoli. Despite the number of Covid-19 laboratories having expanded from five laboratories in four municipalities in May to 15 across eight of Libya's municipalities in August, the increased geographic reach of testing capacity has failed to translate into improved containment strategies. Aside from the dearth in testing, which has hampered efforts to track the spread of the virus, citizens' unwillingness to comply with containment procedures and curfews has also catalyzed the proliferation of cases.[3]

War", *The New Humanitarian*, June 2020.

[2] *Libya Coronavirus: 5,232 Cases And 113 Deaths - Worldometer, Worldometers Info*, September 2020.

[3] Health Sector Libya, "Libya: Health Sector Bulletin (July 2020)", *reliefweb*, August 2020.

Yet, despite its increasingly devastating socio-economic and health impact, Libyans' experience with Covid-19 has unfolded almost in a world of its own, barely impacting the Libyan civil war and its dynamics. Instead, civilians across the country bear the brunt of the virus' spread as authorities governing their areas fail to govern and usher in an appropriate public health response. Ominously, the spread of the pandemic has also occurred against the backdrop of an unprecedented internationalization of the Libyan conflict, with foreign powers more directly involved in driving the conflict than ever before. However, instead of triggering a concerted diplomatic effort to bring an end to the protracted violence, the concomitance of the virus' spread with the globalization of the "civil" war has compounded Western indifference towards the North African country and undermined prospects for a peaceful resolution of its citizens' plight. As a global black swan event, the pandemic has also exacerbated domestic and international actors' tendency to pursue policy choices driven by self-interest and zero-sum calculations at the expense of local populations. The result is, quite literally, the war equivalent of a *tragedy of the commons*, a scenario in which neither Libya's political elite nor their proxy backers are likely to win, but where Libyans definitely lose as disease and violence ravages their country.

Western Indifference, Oil Politics and Covid-19

The internationalization of Libya's war since the launch of Khalifa Haftar's offensive beginning 4 April 2020 on the Tripoli-based Government of National Accord (GNA) has had an impact on the ability and willingness of Libya's authorities to respond to the pandemic. The surprise offensive, green-lit by Washington[4] and launched days before a UN-brokered Libyan national conference was organized, has placed Libya at the center of several overlapping geopolitical rivalries. Western complacency

---

[4] D. Kirkpatrick, "The White House Blessed A War In Libya, But Russia Won It", *The New York Times*, 14 April 2020.

in the face of a potential Libyan relapse into authoritarianism under Haftar betrayed a degree of duplicity permeating the foreign policy apparatus of most Western countries. The failure to condemn the attack – let alone act against it – provided Turkey the opportunity to exert disproportionate leverage on the GNA, which it intervened to protect against Haftar, and more importantly, the United Arab Emirates (UAE). Moscow also capitalized on the West's indifference to scale up its military presence in Libya by transferring jets and mercenaries to support the LAAF.[5] In this kaleidoscopic landscape, Covid-19 is but an added layer of complexity that – while having devastating impact on Libya's socio-economic conditions – has not tapered the forces driving its conflict.

The ability of Libya's domestic actors to pursue their zero-sum calculations and drive their own country to ruin in the process has been afforded by the unabated military support which they have received from their international backers. The outbreak of Covid-19 has not diminished this trend, contributing instead to its exacerbation. Overall, the pandemic was, by and large, perceived as a window of opportunity by proxy powers, one which they sought to utilize to advance their foreign policy agenda against their adversaries in Libya. Indeed, even while Libya's main proxy meddlers – such as the UAE, Turkey, and Russia – were domestically grappling with the virus' spread, they significantly escalated their foreign-operated airstrikes as well as their transfers of weapons and mercenaries to Libya. Yet, despite Libya's military and political spheres gradually becoming the battleground for these meddlers to settle scores, they preferred direct intervention over propping up the capabilities of their local allies.[6] In that sense, while the dimensions and manifestations of the Libyan conflict grew more international,[7]

---

[5] U.S. Department of Defense – AFRICOM, *Russia, Wagner Group Continue Military Involvement In Libya*, July 2020.
[6] E. Badi, "Covid-19 and Proxy Conflict: The Case of Libya", *Proxy Wars Initiative*, May 2020.
[7] W. Lacher, *The great carve-up: Libya's internationalised conflicts after Tripoli*, SWP

this did not translate into improved governance capabilities or a better public health response by domestic parties, which prioritized the war effort instead.

In addition, the global economic downturn that the pandemic has spurred, coupled with a drop in global oil prices, has also affected the behavior of local and international actors in the Libyan theater. Foreign meddlers ironically intensified their interventionism in Libya at the same time they experienced a surge of cases and were confronted with economic woes back home. Depending on their geostrategic calculations and perceived opportunity costs, foreign actors disregarded the financial burden of their involvement or the reputational risks their actions may engender. For instance, the Turkish lira's depreciation did not act as a deterrent for Turkey's military entrenchment in Western Libya, a momentum which grew more apparent after the GNA's capture of Wutiya airbase in late May. Similarly, in July, the UAE – conspiring with Moscow – also wilfully disrupted a US-backed deal that would have seen Haftar's six-month long blockade on Libyan oil exports lifted.[8] In other words, the pandemic prompted middle powers to capitalize on Western indifference to pursue expansionism; a policy choice achieved at the expense of Libya's socio-economic wellbeing. This further hampered the ability to coordinate a public health response, putting the onus on Libya's divided, corrupt, feeble, and contending governing authorities to organize it themselves.

Dysfunctional and Divided Response

The confluence of these geopolitical calculations played into Libyan parties' decision to shun German efforts to broker a ceasefire following the Libya-related Berlin Summit of January 2020. The United Nations' Secretary General appeal

---

Berlin, June 2020.
[8] "Libya's NOC accuses UAE of being behind oil blockade", *Reuters*, 12 July 2020.

for a global ceasefire to help unite efforts to fight Covid-19 in vulnerable countries in early March also fell on deaf ears. Instead, both the Government of National Accord (GNA) and authorities in eastern Libya – the House of Representatives, the Interim Government, and the LAAF – attempted to put in place curfews, closed educational institutions, and launched modest awareness campaigns to encourage social distancing in their respective areas of control, preferring a dysfunctional and divided response over a nationally-coordinated effort.

In Western Libya, the GNA was swift to create a US$358 million fund to combat the outbreak in March, but it did not specify where it would spend the funds, nor did it outline a viable crisis management plan. The LAAF securitized the response to the pandemic by creating a Covid-19 committee headed by figures aligned with Khalifa Haftar, including his chief of staff. The LAAF committee was more concerned with stifling criticism over shortcomings in the public health response than with containing the spread.[9] However, in their attempts to compartmentalize their divided public health response from their respective mobilization for war, these actors undermined the former while prioritizing the latter. Perhaps no image captures the contradiction better than one taken by Egyptian-Canadian photographer Ammru Salahuddien, which shows a GNA fighter in Tripoli's frontline holding his rifle while wearing a surgical mask. In line with the tragedy of the commons, domestic parties, egged on by their international backers, pursued narrow self-interests, inadvertently self-sabotaging their own country in the process.

In many respects, the pandemic has become merely another facet of Libya's conflict. Across the Libyan territory are various vulnerable populations, not in the least citizens in Western Libya, particularly those in Tripoli. Others vulnerable segments of society include migrants, refugees, IDPs, women, and

---

[9] F. Wehrey, *Libya And Coronavirus - Coronavirus In Conflict Zones: A Sobering Landscape*, Carnegie Endowment for International Peace, 14 April 2020.

children, all of which have faced several constraints in their ability to take precautionary measures against the virus owing to the ongoing war. Between 1 January and 30 June 2020, the United Nations Support Mission in Libya (UNSMIL) has documented hundreds of civilian casualties due to airstrikes, ground clashes, and shelling. Eighty percent of these casualties have been attributable to the LAAF, with many civilian returnees dying from the explosion of landmines left by Haftar's forces and Russian mercenaries before they retreated from Tripoli's suburbs towards Sirte and Jufra in June of 2020.[10] Explosive ordinance has constrained citizens' ability to access basic supplies and services, but also severely hampered humanitarian organizations attempting to reach Libya's at-risk populations. The geographic expansion of the conflict towards Tarhuna, and subsequently towards Sirte, has also generated waves of IDPs that are highly vulnerable to an outbreak.

More broadly, health facilities in both LNA and GNA-held territories lack the human and technical capacity to deal with the contemporary outbreak, with testing capabilities limited across the country as cases soared in July. In keeping with its track record of abysmal governance, the GNA mismanaged the crisis response, appointing notoriously corrupt figures with no public health background to contain the spread. Moreover, lack of medical equipment at hospitals due to protracted import restrictions has also led to some medical staff boycotting their shifts at hospitals in fear of contracting the virus. Health infrastructure has also not been spared the effects of war: on 7 April 2020, Al Khadra Hospital, a 400-bed facility in Tripoli that was tasked with treating Covid-19, was momentarily evacuated due to shelling by Haftar's LAAF.[11] Indeed, the latter seemingly weaponized global preoccupation with the pandemic to scale up attacks on civilian suburbs in Tripoli. This behaviour has also galvanized other armed actors into taking control

---

[10] UNSMIL, *Civilian Casualties Report - 1 April - 30 June 2020*, July 2020.
[11] "Eastern Libyan forces attack Tripoli hospital for second day", *Associated Press*, 7 April 2020.

over utilities as a tool for collective punishment or a means of bargaining. In April 2020, at a time where access to water is the most basic requirement for precautionary measures against Covid-19, a forced closure of the southern pipelines of the Great Man-Made River project by an armed group cut water to over 3 million people in Western Libya.[12]

Much like in other countries, both of Libya's authorities initially announced a suspension of all travel to and from Libya. In practice, the sudden decision left hundreds of Libyan citizens stranded in airports across the world. These citizens were brought home in May through a generously funded – but badly executed – GNA repatriation plan which flew citizens to Libya's East and its West. Soon after, Covid-19 cases began gradually increasing in Northern Libya, and a large cluster of cases was discovered in the Southern city of Sebha in late May. Southern Libya – dubbed the Fezzan – is a historically marginalized region which neither of Libya's authorities possesses genuine legitimacy and control over. Neither the GNA nor the Haftar-aligned authorities focused on identifying virus cases across populations in the Fezzan, and their prioritization of the military build-up in Central Libya *de-facto* prevented the implementation of sustainable lockdowns in their areas of control, let alone in the sparsely populated South. The discovery of Libya's first cluster of Covid-19 cases in Sebha essentially spoke to the dysfunctionality characterizing the country's divided public health response and the tragedy of those at its margins. To make matters worse, instead of prompting Eastern and Western-based authorities to shift course and cooperate on managing the crisis, the event was used as part of pro-LAAF and pro-GNA media outlets' war propaganda campaigns in which each party accuses the opposing one of being responsible for spreading Covid-19 inside the country.

---

[12] "In Libya, water cuts add to misery of conflict and coronavirus", *Reuters*, 8 April 2020.

All in all, Libya's national-level authorities have not passed the litmus test of governance that the Covid-19 crisis has presented. Both have squandered lavish funds while failing to procure testing and medical supplies, let alone devise appropriate containment measures and sustainable lockdown strategies. The lack of transparency that has characterized the securitized response of the LAAF's and GNA's bungled measures has fuelled the spread of destabilizing rumours, a factor which has undermined Libyan citizens' willingness to comply with social distancing measures across the country. Worsening living conditions are exacerbating social discontent, with fuel shortages and daily electricity cuts of more than 15 hours a day also straining the capacity of decaying health facilities.[13] Inflation and lack of liquidity are also forcing prolonged periods of social contact as lines for cash and limited costly basic supplies have become increasingly common. If the spread of the virus is to be contained, it will be by neither the national authorities nor their foreign backers, but by local constituencies and – potentially – decisionmakers and armed groups affiliated with them.

Covid-19 Remodels Local-National Relationships

What is already being witnessed because of the dysfunctional response of national authorities to the virus' spread is a fracturing of the tenuous relationships that existed between a self-serving political elite and local communities. National authorities' failure to govern had almost become an accepted reality across Libya, however, the spread of Covid-19 is not an event the country's populace can merely endure or wait out without reaction. Already, calls to protest governing authorities' abysmal response are gaining traction. Moreover, what is often omitted about the Libyan landscape is that, despite the country's

---

[13] T. Megerisi, "A Libya Story: Pandemic And Human Rights In Times Of Conflict", *Open Democracy*, 4 May 2020.

social fabric having been torn apart by perpetual turmoil, familial bonds are still extremely strong. The fact that Libya's median age is around 28 years means that these bonds will not be spared by Covid-19. Indeed, cases of community spread are likely to increasingly involve young adults acting as pathogen vectors that will infect parents and grandparents. In that sense, higher authorities' incompetent response to the pandemic will represent an affront to family links. In the worst cases, the governments' ineptitude will manifest itself as tragedies that will be felt inside Libyan homes. This will fuel social discontent, catalyzing both the GNA's and the LAAF's loss of legitimacy while communities opt to mobilize independently at the grassroots level to contain the spread. In other words, while bringing the governance and legitimacy deficit of national authorities to light, Covid-19 will also reconfigure relationships between local stakeholders and national authorities, with the former growing more autonomous against the backdrop of the latter's gradual loss of popularity.

How successful this forced devolution of authority is at tapering the spread will depend on several factors, not least being how cohesive the community is in these locales. Indeed, tightly knit communities will likely fare better at collectively committing to social distancing measures and at grassroots mobilization. Depending on the context, this will be organized by local governance units such as municipalities, informal social and tribal councils, or even trusted community leaders. Indeed, these stakeholders' accountability and proximity to their constituencies outmatches that of any national-level structure. Yet, despite their best efforts, Libya's centralized governance paradigm dictates that these actors will be constrained by national authorities' policies anyway. While they may choose to organize locally, they will still depend – to a degree – on resources allocated by the central governments and on the coherence of the policies they adopt. In the best-case scenario, this dependence will prompt these actors to demand mechanisms for better cooperation or distribution of funds from the GNA and the Eastern-based authorities. However, a more likely scenario is that this would prompt a resurgence of localism that would manifest itself as entire cities and towns closing themselves off to the rest of the country while hoarding resources to protect their own constituencies.

Whether the virus' spread triggers coerced decentralization or protectionist localism, the dislocation of linkages between the local and the national level presents an opportunity for Libya's panoply of local armed groups.[14] Indeed, either of these two scenarios would be used for these armed actors to present themselves as essential partners for Covid-19 response, whether by cooperating with national authorities or contending with them. Some of these hybrid armed actors are already redefining their raison d'être as enforcers of curfews, an activity through which they are deriving funds by collecting fines and imposing taxes on merchants transporting equipment through their areas of control. As the crisis protracts, others could leverage the relationship of dependency between them and national authorities to divert resources, medical equipment or worse, obtain official mandates that will grant them special powers and under a veneer of legitimacy which they are likely to retain in the long run. Some of Libya's armed actors in coastal towns will once again reconvert themselves into counter-migration partners, especially as Europe's obsession with deterring migration from Libya is exacerbated by the possibility that migrant populations fleeing the North African country may be carrying the virus. In sum, the spread of Covid-19 in Libya is likely to compound the fragmentation of its atomized security sector regardless of the policies adopted to contain the spread.

---

[14] E. Badi, *Coronavirus in Libya: The Contagion of Instability*, ISPI Commentary, ISPI, 7 May 2020.

Conclusion

Libya's conflict was already an internecine struggle before Covid-19 gripped the North African country and brought its citizens more suffering. As elsewhere in the MENA region and beyond it, the pandemic is laying bare the shortcomings of governing authorities and is aggravating pre-existing political, social, and economic trends. However, nowhere else in the world did the pandemic merely dovetail as an added shade of desolation in an already depressing canvas. The fact that even the real prospect of widespread contagion and pestilence is failing to bring Libya's war to a halt speaks to the extent to which it has become a conflict driven by domestic and international actors that have little to no regards for the needs and aspirations of the country's own citizens. Egged on by opportunistic proxy meddlers, Libya's political elite has once again abdicated its responsibility to govern in favour of plundering state coffers and pushing for war. However, in pursuing cynical machinations driven by zero-sum calculations, they are rendering themselves irrelevant to their international backers while losing whatever negligible social legitimacy they possessed amongst local constituencies.

The result is an idiosyncratic situation – a war-equivalent of a *tragedy of the commons* – where Libya's proxy meddlers drive the country to ruin as they intervene to prolong an unwinnable war their local allies have become insignificant to. Ironically, by wilfully wasting the opportunity to devise functionable policies to address the spread of the virus, Libya's competing national authorities are also becoming irrelevant to governance altogether. While the flawed public health response to the pandemic is in line with Libyan authorities' abysmal track record in service provision and crisis management, the social and economic fallout from the virus' spread on Libya's society is likely to force some change in governance. Depending on the locale, this will either force decentralization or trigger protectionist localism – both processes which Libya's wide array of armed actors will seek to capitalize on. In a twisted turn of events, the pandemic's similar devastating effects across the Libyan territory will highlight that the entirety of the country suffers from structural deficiencies, an event that will challenge the long-running idea that partitioning the North African state may resolve its long-standing tribulations. Nevertheless, brought together by the shared misery inflicted upon them by proxy powers and institutional sclerosis, Libyans will have no choice but to disrupt the *status quo*.

2. Algeria: Politics and Protests in Coronavirus Times

Yahia Mohamed Lamine Mestek

Algeria confirmed the first case of Covid-19 within its borders in late February when it was declared that the virus was imported by an Italian citizen who arrived in the country on 17 February 2020 and later placed in isolation. A month later, officials suspended non-cargo domestic and international air and maritime travel and closed all universities, schools, kindergartens, and mosques. Importantly, officials banned the demonstrations held each Friday since 22 February 2019.

In addition to these measures, the Algerian government has followed the recommendations of the World Health Organization (WHO) thenceforth to reduce the spread of Covid-19. Algeria was one of the first countries in the region to close its borders and implement partial lockdowns and curfew measures in critical areas such as Algiers, Blida, Batna, Oran, TiziOuzou, Setif and many other cities with highest number of Covid-19 cases. The state also used mass media to spread awareness.

At the current stage of the pandemic at the time of writing, Algeria is ranked eighth in the MENA region, with 0.062% of the population affected thanks to decisive measures that have limited contagion thus far. Many observers associate this low rate with Algeria's young population (70% are under 30 years old), given that youth tend to face lower risks in terms of the health impact of the Covid-19. However, despite the fact that hospital capacity is increasing and there is a 68.1% recovery rate, Algeria has ranked second after Egypt in the MENA region for Covid-19 deaths, with a 3.9% mortality rate.

The following chapter will analyze the outcomes of Covid-19 in Algeria by illustrating the growing complexity of its interplay with the Algerian regime and the *Hirak* mass protest movement, which is believed to be the only real opposition.[1] It will demonstrate the political impact of the pandemic on the political transition; then proceed with an exploration of the effect on the socio-economic situation in Algeria. To achieve the chapter's objective, micro-level and multi-variables analysis were adopted to look at all aspects of the subject.

The Political Impact of Covid-19 on Algeria

Since its beginning, the pandemic has paved the way for the Algerian regime to control the *Hirak*. After the government's decree prohibiting the protest movement, nominally to prevent the spread of the pandemic, some key figures in the protest saw the move as a convenient attempt to restrict the demonstrations. *Hirak* decided to mobilize virtually, especially on Facebook and YouTube, where people began going live or using memes and videos to denounce the government's inefficiency. The regime responded by using local oppression, arresting activists under the guise of enforcing the law, especially Article 144 Bis from the Algerian penal code, which punishes any "offenses" or "insults" against the President and public official with imprisonment or fines of 1,000-500,000 Algerian dinars, a prohibitive sum in the country.[2]

---

[1] During the last twenty years of former President Abdelaziz Bouteflika's reign, the "opposition" parties largely embraced the regime for survival. With no real opposition, Bouteflika followed what could be called a "corruption democratization policy" with the complicity of some foreign countries. To minimize the influence of his political opposition, Bouteflika created more than 67 new parties, supporting them financially while exploiting their internal problems and undemocratic structures to ensure their loyalties. This was not a true democracy, by any standards.

[2] Penal Code (promulgated by Order No. 66-156 of 18 Safar 1386

The regime has already jailed demonstrators and journalists who spoke out against "Le Pouvoir" and its figures, such as the President. It is notable that while 10,000 prisoners have been released by the President, 75 of whom were prisoners of conscience, many new individuals from the protest movement have been arrested and put in jail during the pandemic, and some personalities of the *Hirak* see that as a play by the government to contain the virtual demonstration and put the opposition in check.

The main impact of Covid-19 on the Algerian political scene has manifested in the difficulty to return to physical demonstrations, giving the authorities time to catch their breath.

However, it looks like the President may have the goodwill to respond to the demands of the *Hirak*, but the pandemic has slowed down all political reforms, especially those related to changing the constitution and challenging the political-economical elites. To reach a consensual constitution, the executives shared the constitutional draft with all the actors (political parties and key figures, civil society, and the public opinion). A debate has opened during the lockdown. Many declared that this draft does not reflect the new Algerian ambitions and intentions, dismissing it as a continuation of the current constitution drafted by former President Abdelaziz Bouteflika.

More than 2,500 remarks and recommendations have been addressed to the Constitutional Committee that prepared the new draft constitution. On 8 January, and less than two weeks after he took power, the Algerian President appointed a constitutional committee of 17 experts in constitutional law, headed by former UN expert Ahmed Araba, to conduct a comprehensive review of the new constitution and reformulate it to build what he calls "the new Algeria." As of September

corresponding to 8 June 1966) https://ihl-databases.icrc.org/applic/ihl/ihl-nat.nsf/0/2C7A71B74DFAB0EBC1256DCF005B4C6B.

2020, the draft constitutional reforms were adopted by Algeria's Parliament and will be put to referendum on 1 November, the anniversary of the start of Algeria's war of independence from France.[3]

Democracy is a balance of power between the state and the people. Algeria is no exception to that rule, and recently the struggle was defined between the regime and the *Hirak*. This is an unbalanced situation since the *Hirak* is not an institution, and the regime on the other hand owns all the institutions. For this reason, the *Hirak* will not win any other rights unless it becomes an institution.

Historically, all Algerian movements, namely those of October 1988, April 2001, and the Arab Spring in 2011, had a central leadership, a structure, and a political project. All of them were absorbed by the regime. Thus, in the public consciousness, the idea comes to mind that if the *Hirak* were to put forth a central leadership, they too would be coopted.

This is a double-edged sword. The absence of a central leadership or a pivotal force, which would determine the *Hirak*'s reaction to the regime's policies internally and externally *ipso facto,* is the reason for the movement's failure to gain more rights. These weaknesses in the *Hirak* (a movement without a leader, structure, or defined political project) have also helped the regime to reach cohesion and respond in the face of demands.

The popular movement's fate is governed by several variables. These variables are:[4]

1. The outbreak of the Covid-19 pandemic put an end to public gatherings and demonstrations, at the behest of the regime, a year after the mass rallies started in February 2019. However, with the increasing severity of Covid-19 casualties, the popular movement's conviction grew that preventing gatherings is not only a

---

[3] "Algerian Parliament adopts draft constitutional reforms", *Al Jazeera*, 20 September 2020.
[4] W.A. al-Hay, *Strategic Situation Assessment: The Prospects of Algerian Policy Between Change and Adaptation*, Al-Zaytouna Center, July 2020, pp. 19-20.

political "move" to control the movement, but rather an objective necessity. Accordingly, the regime's success in confronting the pandemic might serve to enhance its legitimacy and limit the *Hirak* movement. However, its failure might exacerbate political and socio-economic grievances, which would open the way for the *Hirak* movement to return, but less regularly, although there might be a fracture within the movement between those who may "risk" organizing protests and those whose concerns regarding the pandemic prevent them from participating.

2. The confrontations between the regime and the *Hirak* movement in 2019 were generally peaceful. The compliance of the regime with several demands, such as the exclusion of Bouteflika and the imprisonment of some figures symbolic of the regime's corruption (despite the arrest of some activists and leaders within the movement), has enabled the authorities to strengthen political stability, which it ultimately failed to do during the Black Decade.

3. There are weaknesses in the *Hirak* movement and corresponding advantages enjoyed by the regime, including:
    — The absence of a central leadership or a pivotal force that determines the movement's reaction toward the regime's policies internally and externally.
    — The consensus of political visions within the regime: when there was a clash of factions within the Algerian system, the *Hirak* movement was able to achieve many of its demands.
    — The escalation of regional concerns (especially the Libyan crisis), which might push the *Hirak* to wait for the outcome of the Libyan developments. This trend might expand if proxy wars escalate in Libya.
    — Some fractures in the *Hirak* movement, which have manifested during the demonstrations. These rifts are driven in part by arguments between subcultures

and around identity. For example, there is continuous debate about *Amazigh* identity, with significant variation in estimating their population and the limits on expressing cultural identity, such as arrests of some who raised *Amazigh* flags at protests. Amazigh people are present in public institutions, where reports indicate their high percentage in the technocratic sectors, but they have less influence in the military and security institutions, especially after the change in military intelligence. The acceptance of the *Amazigh* language varies: it is constitutionally accepted, though socially, it is less accepted. Identifying it as a national language or an official language is also a topic of debate within the *Hirak*.

Now Algeria is at a crossroads. The government must either take the risk to empower the *Hirak* and coopt it into the political system or keep it politically weak. In a recent article, Dalia Ghanem declares that the Algerian regime has shown a significant degree of resilience and adaptability during upheavals;[5] this will likely continue.

Despite the mass protest movement and the last presidential election, the People's National Army still dominates the country. This order will likely continue for the foreseeable future. In assessing adaptation by the Algerian regime, Prof. Walid Abd al-Hay found that between 1962 and 2020 the military has comprised the presidency 58.3% of the time, while civilians have governed 41.7% of the same period. It is noteworthy that most of the civilian periods were transitional periods, which were unable to establish stability, allowing the military leadership to be more sustainable.[6]

However, international competition in the region, turmoil in Libya, and persistent tensions to the south of Algeria, especially

---

[5] D. Ghanem, *Limiting Change Through Change: The Key to the Algerian Regime's Longevity*, Carnegie Middle East Center, May 2018.
[6] W.A. al-Hay (2020), p. 18.

in Mali and Niger, might force the regime to pursue the choice of army interference abroad. Moreover, security threats in the country's neighborhood, even without Algerian intervention, keep Algerian decisions in the hand of the military and other security forces and seemingly justifies military spending to the public.[7]

Algeria ranks third globally in terms of the ratio of military spending to GDP, reaching 5.3%. Military spending represents 13.8% of the Algerian government's expenditures. Between 2010 and 2020, the average annual military spending rate is about US$9.6 billion. With expenditure vacillating due to fluctuating oil and gas prices, the current government decided to reduce its spending by 9%.[8] Despite this, the country's security apparatus will likely remain strong.

The Impact of Covid-19 on the Algerian Socio-Economic Situation

The economic impact of Covid-19 on Algeria is relevant to explain the interplay between the Algerian regime and the mass protest movement. The words of a famous Algerian aptly sum up the impact of economic downturn on the *Hirak*: "Starve the dog and it'll follow you". During the pandemic, many Algerian people, especially those working in the black market, which represents around 25% of the Algerian economy, lost their jobs, and the regime capitalizes on that by giving them financial aid. The regime continues this policy with some industries and small businesses, and 2,795 artists benefit from this aid. The government sent many solidarity convoys to carry food supplies destined for needy families living in remote areas and *Bedouin* (nomadic) areas, as well as to people with special needs. These measures will enable the regime to strengthen its political stability in the short term.

---

[7] Ibid.
[8] Ibid, p. 3.

However, challenges loom. Oil and gas are the backbone of the Algerian economy, and many global economic institutions foresee stormy days ahead due to the sharp and continuous decline in the prices of oil. The World Bank's last report on the Algerian economic situation declared that the Covid-19 outbreak would slow down consumption and investment while falling oil prices cut into fiscal and export revenues. The new government faces a difficult task maintaining macroeconomic stability, responding to the public health crisis, and pursuing structural reforms.[9]

The present government has the will to liberate the Algerian economy from the control of the energy sector. Nevertheless, Algeria shows a total dependency on hydrocarbons; 95% of its revenues depend on its exports of "black gold". Algeria's foreign exchange reserves have measured at US$53.6 billion in June 2020, compared to US$55.2 billion in the previous month.[10]

The deterioration of vital Algerian economic sectors has accelerated since the outbreak of Covid-19; hydrocarbons recorded a drop of 3.3%. Mines and quarries show a decrease of 4.8%. Metal, mechanical and electrical industries have seen a decrease of 38.2%. Agro-Food Industries registered an increase of 5.9% in the first quarter of 2020, a positive rate, but inferior to those observed in the previous quarter (+11.3%). Building Materials continued their downward trend and showed a negative variation of -11.5%. Chemical industries observe a drop of 11.5%. Textile industries record a negative variation of -14.6%. The Wood and Paper industries observe a drop of 23.3% in the first quarter of 2020.[11]

The scene becomes further complicated if we add the decline of the economic growth rate, which started in 2015 (the rate was about 3.5%), and in 2023, it is expected to reach 0.5%, as shown in the following graph:

---

[9] The World Bank, *Algeria's Economic Outlook*, April 2020.
[10] Algeria Foreign Exchange Reserves, CEIC, June 2020.
[11] Indice de la production industrielle. Au 1er trimester 2020 (Industrial production index) - in Q1 2020, no. 892, June 2020.

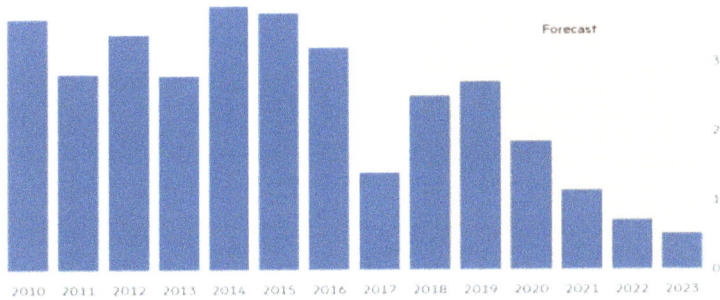

Source: W. A. al-Hay. *Strategic Situation Assessment: The Prospects of Algerian Policy Between Change and Adaptation*. July 2020 p 11.

Besides, the World Bank report announces that Algeria is facing a combined shock from halving oil prices, a public health crisis, and global economic disruptions following the Covid-19 outbreak. An oil price at US$30/barrel in 2020 would decrease Algeria's total fiscal revenues by 21.2%. Despite cuts to public investment (-9.7%) and public consumption (-1.6%) envisaged by the 2020 Finance Law, the fiscal deficit would increase to 16.3% of GDP. Meanwhile, the sharp decline in export revenues (-51%) will lead the trade deficit to expand to 18.2% of GDP and the current account deficit to peak at 18.8% of GDP in 2020, despite the regime's efforts to contain imports and weaken domestic demand.[12]

The post-pandemic economic consequences on the Algerian regime's stability and resilience represent an opportunity for the *Hirak* movement to regain the street. Further, the openness of the regime to create new political, economic, and social elite could bring the *Hirak* into the official institutions.

While acknowledging the importance of the economic impact of Covid-19 on Algeria, the social impact also has an

---

[12] The World Bank (2020), p. 1.

essential role in defining the interplay between the Algerian regime and the *Hirak* mass protest movement.

The increase of violence correlated to the economic situation reveals the extent of the threat to Algerian society. Official statistics indicate an increase in Algeria's crime rate during the first half of the year 2020, recording a quarter of a million crimes, with an average of 693 accidents per day, in which more than 220,000 people were involved. The statistics consider 70,000 cases of violent crimes against women. The statistics mention that unemployed people are at the forefront of those implicated in the crimes. The demographics associated with these crimes also indicate economic factors: 3.8% of those who committed recorded crimes were under the age of 18, 57.3% were between 18 and 30 years old, 25.63% were between 30 and 40 years old, and those over the age of 40 exceeded 13%. The gender distribution was estimated at 97.8% male, and 2.20% female.[13]

Moreover, during the Covid-19 pandemic, Algeria witnessed an increase in domestic violence as well as divorce rates. Official statistics show that 20% of marriages end in divorce and that the divorce to marriage ratio has increased dramatically since 2014, reaching more than 68,000 divorce cases annually at a rate of one case every 8 minutes. This could be caused in part by increased economic and political pressures, leading to social unrest with divorce and domestic violence as a prominent manifestation.[14]

Social turmoil indirectly nourishes political turmoil, and vice versa. This may indirectly impact the Algerian regime's grip on power. Furthermore, the *Hirak* movement can continue to challenge the regime by increasing its demands and criticizing its performance, especially since the economic crisis is at the door.

---

[13] A. Yahya, "700 crimes a day in Algeria and society is at risk", *Independent Arabia*, July 2020.
[14] Ibid.

Conclusion

It seems that the Algerian internal conditions (political, economic, and social), as we described, lead to thinking in two prospects: short term and long term.

In the short term, the regime has to choose from four courses of action: whether it retains power or returns it to the *Hirak* movement, and whether it acquiesces or resists the expansion of political participation. Each option, however, imposes costs on the military and the political system.

1. **Progressive-return and Restrict:** The regime can progressively return power to the *Hirak* movement through purging government officials and pushing new groups to political power by nomination into office or elections.

2. **Semi-return and Expand:** The regime can semi-return power to the *Hirak* movement and permit the previous political groups which were blocked to come to power under new conditions (i.e. political and economic reconciliation).

3. **Retain and Restrict:** The regime can retain power and continue to resist the *Hirak* movement's expansion through political participation. In this case, despite whatever intentions the regime may have, they will inevitably be driven to more repressive measures.

4. **Retain and Expand:** the regime can retain power and permit or, indeed, capitalize upon the expansion of political participation to the *Hirak* movement.

In the long run, options three and four will reinforce the fears of the regime's longevity *ad vitam aeternam*. Based on the previous factors, option one will create the trend to "relative" stability in Algeria and a new generation of political and economic forces could take shape within the next 3–5 years to be more responsive to the local, regional and international challenges. Option two would create real stability through a new political, economic, and social pact between old regime figures and the new government, based on new values and conditions. This path would take Algeria to durable stability and create real cohesion among all parts of the regime and society. In this situation, Algeria could become a regional player by exporting its stability toward the Sahel region and Libya. It is possible that the political impact of Covid-19 could be used to transition the country toward a better future.

3. Egypt: The Pandemic Crisis in a Time of Authoritarianism

Hafsa Halawa

Over the last decade, Egypt has witnessed significant political upheaval, resulting in two major political schisms in the social uprising of 2011 and the popularly backed military coup that followed in 2013. The political opening brought about by the removal of reigning strongman President Mohamed Hosni Mubarak in 2011 brought about short-lived but monumental political change and created opportunities for pluralism in politics, a widening of civic space and civil society activity, and freer, more independent media. However, the politics of the Muslim Brotherhood-dominated transition period resulted in societal fear of a perceived shift in the nature of Egypt's identity and widespread discontent both about the nature of the party's brand of leadership and the direction which it was felt the country was moving toward.

The 30 June protests led to the ouster of then-President (and leader of the Muslim Brotherhood's Freedom and Justice Party, FJP) Mohamed Morsi by the military, backed by popular support from the street in the form of mass protests.[1] In the years since July 2013 there has been an unprecedented crackdown on fundamental freedoms, such as expression, assembly, and speech as well as widely documented human rights abuses through the arguably unlawful detention of tens of thousands

---

[1] D.D. Kirkpatrick, "Army Ousts Egypt's President; Morsi Is Taken Into Military Custody", *The New York Times*, 3 July 2013.

of political dissidents and civic activists. The crackdown has also seen a complete closure of political space through years of slow erasure of the thriving pluralism initially created in 2011. The leadership of President (and former Military Field Marshall) Abdel Fattah Al Sisi (2014-present) has gone beyond simply retrenching the decades-long tradition of one-party rule in Egypt.[2] Rather, the leadership of Sisi has pursued control over all state institutions, silencing the judiciary and Parliament into complete submission to the executive and ultimately erasing the "Separation of Powers" principle.[3]

With new challenges presented as of late by the Covid-19 pandemic, President Sisi has sought to absorb even more power, amending instructive legislation to allow the executive branch to gain further legislative and judicial power as well as expanding the administrative control of the state.[4] Covid-19 has effectively provided the context for which Egypt's President can continue to further entrench authoritarian practice and expand toward totalitarianism as the defining feature of his rule.

Egypt's Last Decade:
from Democratic Transition to Military Rule

Following the uprising that led to the removal of Hosni Mubarak from power in 2011, Egypt witnessed a groundswell of civic and political engagement and activity. Over 160 political parties were formed, registering for the country's first post-revolution elections that took place between November 2011 and January 2012.[5] 67 political parties won seats in the election

---

[2] *Egypt under Sisi: From Authoritarian Dominant Party System to Strongman Politics*, JETRO-IDE ME-Review, vol. 6, 2018-2019, pp. 1-3.

[3] *2019 Constitutional Amendments*, Policy Brief, Tahrir Institute for Middle East Policy (TIMEP), 17 April 2019.

[4] Amendments to: Emergency Law 1958 (and amendments); Counterterrorism Laws 2015 (and amendments), Penal Code 1937 (and amendments).

[5] Author's own knowledge as Political Parties Researcher and registered Elections Observer for Egypt's Parliamentary Elections for the National Democratic

for the Lower and Upper Houses of Parliament, through a newly introduced mixed proportional representation list and individual candidacy districts.[6] Over 90% of those parties were deemed newly formed political groups that emerged following the protests that engulfed the country. While the majority of seats belonged to the Islamist Bloc of parties (who had run collectively on the Democratic Front list and included a collective group of Salafi political parties as well as the FJP), an array of political thought was reflected in the eclectic Parliament. Self-identified centrists, leftists, Islamists, socialists, and even "former regime" politicians represented Egypt's first, and only, genuine democratic effort.

The presidential elections that ensued a year later had, at their peak, 14 candidates from all parts of the political spectrum, including representatives of the Mubarak regime and Political Islamists (Muslim Brotherhood and other groups).[7] The first and second rounds of voting in a first-past-the-post system came on either side of a monumental decision from the Supreme Constitutional Court to dissolve the elected Lower House of Parliament.[8] The court's decision was a monumental blow to the democratic transition, despite being cheered by more centrist MPs and supposed liberals. It also impacted the decision-making of voters in the presidential election, left at the final stage to choose between Mubarak's last Prime Minister and former Air Commander Ahmed Shafiq, or the FJP leader and senior member of the Muslim Brotherhood's Guidance Bureau, Mohamed Morsi. The result was a heavily contested election, barely won in the end by FJP leader Morsi.[9]

Institute (July 2011 - February 2012).

[6] *Final Report of the Carter Center Mission to Witness the 2011-12 Parliamentary Elections in Egypt*, Carter Center, August 2012.

[7] T. Plofchan, "Candidates in the 2012 Egyptian Presidential Election", *The Cairo Review*, 27 April 2012.

[8] "Egypt's supreme court dissolves parliament and outrages Islamists", *The Guardian*, 14 June 2012.

[9] D.D. Kirkpatrick, "Named Egypt's Winner, Islamist Makes History", *The New York Times*, 24 June 2012.

The vote itself was mired in controversy. The FJP/MB had deployed tens of thousands of polling agents to every single one of Egypt's 16,0000 poll stations to observe the vote and ballot counting.[10] As a result, the FJP declared victory over a week before the official decision came from the Presidential Elections Committee, ultimately politicizing the entire democratic exercise and putting in doubt the genuine result. The contest left a sour taste in the mouths of political opponents to the MB, with civic activists feeling betrayed and no political representative in the highest office. The election acted to effectively kill off initial hopes that either a non-Islamist or non-regime politician could yield political power in the country.

Throughout the period from Morsi's inauguration until protests once again removed a president from power exactly a year later, Egypt continued to demonstrate and exercise political pluralism, albeit less effectively than during the immediate post-2011 transition. Opposition grew – within both political and civic spaces – over the activity and decision-making of the sitting president, including attempts to subvert the constitution and declare the executive immune from oversight.[11] As a result, violent protests began to emerge between political actors or those they represented, eroding the pluralistic gains made.[12] Slowly but surely, dependence on the military institution became more evident until it reached a fever pitch in June 2013, with citizens actively calling for a return to military rule. On 3 July 2013, then Defense Minister Abdel Fattah Al Sisi addressed the public, stating that the military had removed President Morsi in a bloodless coup, and announcing a roadmap for an alleged transition.[13]

---

[10] *EISA Election Witnessing Mission Report*, Electoral Institute for Sustainability in Africa (EISA), Egypt: Presidential Elections Report no. 45, 2013.

[11] "English text of Morsi's Constitutional Declaration", *Ahram Online*, 22 November 2012.

[12] "Egypt: The Constitutional Declaration and the Spiraling Violence in Egypt that Leads the Country Away from the Path to Democracy", *Euromed Rights*, 6 December 2012.

[13] "Egyptian army suspends constitution and removes President Morsi – as it happened", *The Guardian*, 3 July 2013.

Instead of renewed democratic transition, however, the removal of the MB from power saw tens of thousands arrested as political prisoners and thousands more forced to flee the country, their assets and finances seized by the state.[14] The crackdown on all forms of freedom began almost as soon as Morsi was removed, as the military and other security forces (military police, central security forces, state security, etc.) clashed with civilian protestors who opposed the coup. The stand-off culminated in the largest one-day massacre of civilians the country has arguably ever seen, as up to (and possibly more than) 1,000 protestors were killed on 14 August 2013, with the clearing of protests in squares in central and north Cairo districts.[15]

Following the removal of Political Islamists from power and any form of political life, interim President Adly Mansour (largely believed to have been acting on behalf of current President Sisi at the time), outlawed the entire organization and passed emergency legislation equating Political Islam with terrorism. This was quickly followed by reams of legislation that banned any protest gatherings,[16] declared almost all state institutions military institutions (and thus subject to military jurisdiction and laws),[17] and allowed police access to public and private institutions such as banks and universities.[18] New laws were also drafted to institutionalize years-long security management

---

[14] Z. Laub, *Egypt's Muslim Brotherhood*, Council on Foreign Relations, last updated 15 August 2019.

[15] *The Weeks of Killing, State Violence, Communal Fighting and Sectarian Attacks in the Summer of 2013*, Egyptian Initiative for Personal Rights (EIPR), 14 June 2014.

[16] "Egypt: President Approves Anti-Protest Law", *Library of Congress*, Global Legal Monitor 13 December 2013.

[17] S. Aziz, *The Expanding Jurisdiction of Egypt's Military Courts*, Carnegie Endowment for International Peace, 12 October 2016.

[18] E. Hamed, "Egyptians divided over police presence on university campuses", *Al-Monitor*, 16 April 2014.

of civil society,[19] block the receipt of foreign funding,[20] and expand active cases against foreign and local NGOs, ensnaring dozens and then hundreds of civic actors.[21] Many high-profile civilian activists were also arrested and jailed.[22]

By the time President Sisi came to power officially through elections in 2014, Egypt's democratic reversal was well under way. Since then, however, the crackdown has taken on prolonged and more severe forms. The "disappearing" of individuals has become a common practice by security forces in a country where detention is the main tactic against dissent.[23] Hundreds of NGOs have been forced to close owing to lack of resources or pressure from security forces, as they create a climate of fear once again. Thousands of political activists now languish in pre-trial detention,[24] while senior FJP/MB figures are dying in prison[25]. Political parties have either dissolved themselves, fearful of the security crackdown, or have been silenced into submission by the ruling regime.[26] The Judiciary has lost almost all of its independence and ability to challenge the regime due to

---

[19] *Proposed Government Law Makes NGOs Subordinate to Security and Ministry Control,* Egyptian Initiative for Personal Right (EIPR), Press Release, 9 July 2014.

[20] R. Gehad, "Egypt amends penal code to stipulate harsher punishments on foreign funding", *Ahram Online*, 23 September 2014.

[21] Miller and M. Suter, *Case No. 173: The State of Egypt's NGOs*, Atlantic Council, 29 March 2016.

[22] *Timep Brief: Case 173: Egypt's Foreign Funding Case*, Tahrir Institute for Middle East Policy (TIMEP), 28 February 2019.

[23] R. Trafford and M. Ramadhani, "Ruling by fear: Egyptian government 'disappears' 1,840 people in just 12 months", *The Independent*, 10 March 2016.

[24] A. Mikhail, "Interpreting Egypt's Pretrial Detention Laws", *Lawfare*, 10 November 2015.

[25] Senior MB leaders who have died while in detention since 2013 include: former Supreme Guide Mehdi Akef (2017), former President Mohamed Morsi (2019), senior leader and MP Essam el Erain (2020). Senior MB leaders who have died while in detention since 2013 include: former Supreme Guide Mehdi Akef (2017), former President Mohamed Morsi (2019), senior leader and MP Essam el Erain (2020).

[26] M. Dunne and A. Hamzawy, *Egypt's Secular Political Parties: A Struggle for Identity and Independence*, Carnegie Endowment for International Peace, 31 March 2017.

constitutional amendments that have removed such modalities from the institution.[27] Parliament has become an institution that is socially mocked and politically inept, reinstated through elections in late 2015 only to provide a legislative mask for President Sisi's practices, seen as more of way to placate the international community than any sort of commitment to democratization.[28]

Meanwhile, Egypt has suffered socially and economically. An economic crisis that came with the political upheaval forced a significant concession to the international community, resulting in the approval of a US$12 billion IMF (International Monetary Fund) agreement.[29] The result has seen subsidies lifted, the currency devalued by over half, and income wealth destroyed.[30] Consumer spending remains low, inflation has tripled effectively since 2016, and ordinary Egyptians struggle under the weight of financial burdens. Meanwhile, military companies flood the private sector, unfairly competing with civilian companies and foreign investment to gain access to Egypt's riches.

Egypt and Covid-19

On 20 September 2019, a few months before the world would become embroiled in the Covid-19 pandemic, President Sisi witnessed the first genuine social challenge to his leadership since he came to power.[31] Small, short-lived protests swept across

---

[27] *Egypt Constitutional Amendments: Unaccountable Military, Unchecked President and a Subordinated Judiciary*, International Commission of Jurists, April 2019.

[28] S. Hamad, "A cabinet of kleptocracy in Sisi's pseudo-parliament", *The New Arab*, 23 April 2018.

[29] IMF Executive Board Approves US$12 billion Extended Arrangement Under the Extended Fund Facility for Egypt", International Monetary Fund (IMF), Press Release no. 16/501, 11 November 2016.

[30] A. Khafagy, "Celebrating poverty: the IMF in Egypt", *openDemocracy*, 15 November 2019.

[31] "Egyptian authorities threaten to 'decisively confront' protesters", *The Guardian*, 26 September 2019.

a number of cities in Egypt in response to viral claims from a disgruntled military contractor that the military institution and the President were institutionally corrupt. Protests only lasted a few hours and barely managed to gather a few thousand people in each city but sent shockwaves through the country and among the ruling military. In the days that followed, thousands of people were rounded up and detained, including high profile activists who had celebrated the protests online (though no evidence shows they were present themselves), and the security services swarmed city centers setting up checkpoints and stopping citizens at random, primarily to check social media activity on their mobile phones. Private media – once somewhat independent, but nowadays largely owned and coopted by the intelligence and security apparatus – encouraged citizens to alert the police if they encountered dissent in public or online. Independent journalists – already heavily threatened in the country – were targeted, and a significant number were arrested.

However, while the political and civic space was effectively closing prior to the Covid-19 outbreak, Egypt's economy was riding high after a successful 2019.[32] Despite the continued dominance of the military apparatus in the economy, tourism was back to an eight year high,[33] remittances for the year totaled their highest percentage of GDP,[34] large gas discoveries were driving increased oil and gas investment in the country, and international financial experts and investors were excited about the prospects in Egypt.[35]

Much like the rest of the world, Egypt has since been severely impacted by the Covid-19 pandemic and its global and domestic ramifications. The economic fallout has been

---

[32] T. Kaldas, *Egypt's Economy Faces a Double Whammy*, Bloomberg Opinion, 10 March 2020.

[33] M. Maged, "Egypt's tourism saw 21% growth in 2019: UNWTO", *Egypt Independent*, 22 January 2020.

[34] "Egypt Remittances: 2002-2019 Data", Trading Economics.

[35] "S&P positive outlook for Egypt promises new foreign investments in 2020: Moeit", *MENAFN Daily News Egypt*, 12 January 2020.

significant, with tourism reduced to zero and an oil price crash that has jeopardized remittances from the Gulf countries (and Egyptians working abroad), and threatened Egypt's own natural resources market.[36]

It has also come with a significant healthcare toll[37]. The region as a whole has generally emerged from the first phase of the global pandemic with one of the lowest death rates, leading people to draw assumptions related to the young demographic across the MENA region, as well as questions related to climate and possible genetic conditions that could be contributive (albeit all speculative). For its part, Egypt initially benefited generally from a rather "slow curve" of Covid-19 progression across the country, however, the state has been criticized by healthcare specialists for not taking advantage of a relatively contained virus spread at the outset.[38]

Although actual numbers are believed to be much higher, per capita figure comparisons show that Egypt has not suffered the kind of debilitating virus outbreak that other countries in the region, such as Iran or Iraq, have faced. Nevertheless, the outbreak brought with it severe stress on Egypt's healthcare system, and exposed the country's consistently failing bureaucracy.[39] While the global economy slowed to a halt, the country closed its international air space but initially imposed minimal closures of public spaces. As the outbreak progressed, curfew measures and closures of hospitality and green spaces were introduced, as well as specific measures for treatment at hospitals.

---

[36] Egypt's Economy under COVID: Threats and Opportunities", webinar discussion, Middle East Institute, 15 June 2020.

[37] S. Amin, "Pandemic further strains Egypt's dilapidated health system", *Al-Monitor*, 8 April 2020.

[38] "Egypt Faces the Pandemic: Health and Economic Effect", webinar discussion, Carnegie Endowment for International Peace, 11 June 2020.

[39] B. Trew, "'Risk death or risk jail': Health workers around the world detained and attacked during the pandemic", *The Independent*, 19 July 2020.

While the presidency publicly paraded its efforts to support other countries by supplying personal protective equipment (such as the UK, US, Italy, Sudan), doctors slowly began to protest their own lack of equipment and protective measures.[40] Dissent grew among healthcare workers as doctors and other staff began to suffer themselves from the virus, with anger becoming harnessed by the Doctor's Syndicate, formalizing grievances and institutionally challenging the government's response to the pandemic. The government was continually forced to respond to accusations it had left healthcare workers to die, with social debate, religious scholars, and public figures all weighing in on the growing protests from healthcare professionals.[41]

Unsurprisingly, the President was largely absent for large parts of the domestic Covid-19 response. Earlier believed to be suffering himself from the virus,[42] Sisi's absence has since become evidence of a political decision to channel dissent and anger with the domestic Covid-19 response toward the civilian government. As if on cue, as Covid-19 patient numbers swelled and hospitals became overrun, the military – led by President Sisi – announced the opening of a 4,000-bed field hospital created in the heart of Cairo to support the efforts against the virus.[43]

Throughout 2020, as the country battles Covid-19 and the economic hardship that endures as a result, authoritarian measures and practice have only continued. Egypt has already been under continuous Emergency Law provisions since early 2017, however, amendments forced through early on during the

---

[40] "Coronavirus: Egypt sends medical gowns for British health workers", *The National*, 14 April 2020.
[41] J. Rothwell, "Egyptian doctors accused of treason after criticising government's coronavirus response", *The Telegraph*, 8 June 2020.
[42] Interview with retired military official, via skype, March 2020. Interview with retired military official, via skype, March 2020.
[43] "Egypt's Sisi tours Armed Forces medical isolation facilities", *Ahram Online*, 27 June 2020.

pandemic response have seen the President's powers widened at the expense of legal and administrative arms of the state. The President continues to centralize all forms of decision-making and power yielded in the Executive Office, and namely the presidency. As a result, authoritarian practices not only remain omnipresent within society but are becoming harsher still.

A continued crackdown on freedom of expression and speech during the pandemic saw arrests spread from journalists, to female *"TikTok"* users,[44] to a number of healthcare professionals who openly criticized the state response to Covid-19. Doctors were arrested for protesting the lack of protective equipment – refusing to treat Covid-19 patients – following a number of deaths of young doctors from the virus.[45] Beyond the arrests, the state sought to demonize healthcare workers among the general public, invoking some of the country's most senior religious leaders to declare them "murderers" for protesting and refusing to treat patients.[46]

As the country retreated to their homes, prayers were suspended, and mosques were closed. Ramadan iftars and *"taraweeh"* prayers were also cancelled. As citizens retreated from the hustle and bustle of daily life, little was left to occupy them, and as a result social and political issues have since obsessed ordinary citizens. Despite the Covid-19 pandemic and ongoing challenges as depicted by healthcare workers, the country has witnessed a gender-rights revolution in and of itself, as online testimonials of sexual assault have gone viral and expanded, ensnaring a number of institutions and segments of the public.[47] While this particular topic has forced the government to impose new legal conditions on confidentiality

---

[44] "Egypt imprisons female TikTok influencers", *Deutsche Welle*, 29 July 2020.

[45] S. Devi, "Egyptian health workers arrested after Covid-19 comments", *The Lancet*, 8 August 2020.

[46] علي جمعة: قانل فيروس كورونا لغيره قاتل بالتسبب.. فيدي" ("Ali Jumaa: The transmission of the Corona virus to another fought by causing ... my blood"), *Sada Al Balad reporting*, 7 June 2020.

[47] "Is Egypt finally reckoning with sexual assault?", *Al Jazeera*, 14 August 2020.

of victim testimonials, and introduce debate on a draft sexual violence law, the nature of the state is still to confront and crush dissent in all its forms. At least nine women have been arrested for their *TikTok* activity, accused of "debauchery" or "violating public norms and family values". Three women have already been sentenced to up to three years in prison.

Furthermore, the crackdown on the media and journalists continues, with Covid-19 providing no relief in the years-long repression freedom of speech.[48] Meanwhile, the President passes legislation at will, continuing to curb all forms of fundamental freedoms. As well as the Emergency Law amendments passed, amendments to the penal code and the package of counterterrorism laws have also been made while the country is preoccupied with the pandemic.

Entrenching Authoritarianism

Egypt under President Sisi is well known for authoritarian practice and the closure of civic and political space. The Covid-19 pandemic has merely offered the President a new guise within which to pass and enact oppressive legislation that either further entrenches preexisting practices already or introduces new, harsher conditions upon ordinary citizens. As the country adjusts to a slow re-opening of its economy and cautious resumption of normal life, the President fast-tracked legislation and Upper House (Senate) elections in August 2020.[49]

While elections have been a contested but genuine opening for political debate – even under more recent repression – in their various iterations over the last decade, the August 2020 Senate elections were notable only in how they brought back imagery

---

[48] C. MacDiarmid, "Journalist arrested for criticising Egypt's coronavirus response dies after catching it in jail", *The Telegraph*, 14 July 2020.

[49] M. Mourad, "Egyptians vote for newly created Senate", *Reuters*, 11 August 2020.

from the Mubarak era: there was little to no acknowledgement elections were even happening, state TV played reams of film showing citizens in the street celebrating elections, vote-buying featured as a common state-deployed tactic, and apathy largely dominated public response to the elections. The amended laws were also not subject to any judicial or external review, nor was the generally sensitive topic of candidate districts addressed.[50]

That the pandemic has presented new challenges to the state is not to say that this behavior deviates from that which defines this regime, nor that it will continue unimpeded or unchallenged. Egypt's ruling class have reverted to a form of authoritarianism that served Mubarak well for decades, albeit resulting in his eventual removal; however, the current military institution is neither as homogenous as Mubarak's wider leadership was, nor is it as malleable as President Sisi desires.

Propelled by paranoia, genuine cracks have been opening within the military apparatus for years – even before President Sisi came to power. Part of the reasoning behind the authoritarian practice exercised by the Presidency is, in effect, an attempt to put down either rumors or active dissent among both senior military leaders and the lower rank and file of the institution. Over the years the country has witnessed successive public purges of senior military generals, as well as a quieter – almost secretive – string of military court cases against hundreds of young Non-Commissioned Officers (NCOs) believed to oppose President Sisi's agenda.

---

[50] Egypt's electoral laws have hostircally come under severe scrutiny from the SCC over the years, including during the transition period betwen 2011-13. Since President Sisi has come to power, the laws have not faced scrutiny, owing both to the continued reversion to the 2014 presidential elections law that designed districts that remain in place, but also because the Judicial Appointments Law amended by President Sisi in 2017 gave him full authority to designate the makeup of the SCC, resulting in a quiet and pliant court – in contrast to its usual, relatively independent political and juidicial nature.

While President Sisi is clearly a strongman, he does not necessarily enjoy the kind of wholesale support that his predecessors have done, nor has he ever been able to win over complete internal legitimacy for his rise to power. Therefore, means by which to entrench authoritarianism across the country's civilian political space also act to inhibit threats from within the military or broader security apparatus. This has served the President well for a number of years, although it is believed to have been challenged of late, some allege even coinciding with the small civilian protests seen in 2019.[51] More recent legislation passed to prevent any active or retired military officer from running for any form of public office without approval from the most senior military leaders appears to reflect an attempt by the President to curb ambitions within the military, but also to protect his own brand of leadership that has never quite fully consolidated to date.[52]

Conclusion

Egypt has been largely and rightly defined over the last decade for its increased repression, human rights abuses, and primarily the almost complete militarization of civilian way of life, including political and civic rights and activity. Under the leadership that followed the largely pluralistic period between 2011 and 2013, the country has slowly regressed to a position of almost complete political inactivity and unexercised political rights. However, that does not necessarily extend to the general political apathy that defined the majority of the era under former President Hosni Mubarak.

Indeed, the Egyptian citizenry as a whole was awakened by the events of 2011 and continued to openly and actively mobilize for a prolonged period of time, arguably exhausting

---

[51] Interview with Egyptian former official, via skype, May 2020.
[52] "Egypt's Sisi approves ban on retired army officers standing for election", *Reuters*, 29 July 2020.

the public into submission under the threats now posed. There may be little to no room for genuine expression or space to exercise political rights in the current day, but that is not to say that ordinary Egyptian civilians are not politically motivated or have recused themselves from political life.

While there remain only very few who continue to challenge the regime's repression openly through civic engagement and political activity, personal relationships and day-to-day conversations remain highly politicized. The country continues to see individual and collective political expression, and it is reflective of the desire for political representation and rights that only with extreme repression and complete closure of civic and political space has the regime been able to snuff out collective civilian power able to challenge leadership and hold the regime to account.

4. Riding the Pandemic Wave: How the Iraqi Political Elite Survived a Triple Crisis

Abbas Kadhim

I arrived in Baghdad in mid-September 2019 to attend the annual International Energy Forum and conduct routine research and work-related interviews. It was my third visit for the year, and I couldn't help but see the difference in Iraq's capital. For the first time, I was free to come and go to and from my hotel, inside the Green Zone, without the inconvenience of special permits and complicated security arrangements. Concrete barriers were almost completely removed, checkpoints were friendlier and hassle-free, and friends were even able to visit me in the hotel. None of this was possible during my stay at the same hotel just four months earlier. Outside the Green Zone, we enjoyed long restaurant gatherings with old friends and new acquaintances until past mid-night. On the business side, it was the first time where the only conferences in Baghdad were not on terrorism, but economics and reconstruction and it was the first post-2003 summer that Iraq had no demonstrations against shortages in electricity supply.

Iraq was moving on a very promising trajectory, and international confidence in the country's potential was steadily coming back. A major agreement was prepared to change the paradigm of Iraqi reconstruction projects, where a great deal of corruption was committed. For more than a decade, billions of US dollars were allocated to projects that were done on paper only – some projects were done twice in this fashion, while the money went in the pockets of corrupt officials and their political entities. To curb this practice, Prime Minister Adil Abdul-Mahdi planned a new system: "oil for reconstruction". For this ambitious undertaking, the government signed several memoranda of understanding with China and established a fund where oil proceeds are deposited and used to pay for future reconstruction projects by various Chinese companies.

However, three major crises took the country by storm: a wave of widespread protests that were accompanied by a level of violence unprecedented in the post-2003 era, a lethal escalation in the US-Iranian conflict that was fought on Iraqi soil, and a worldwide raging pandemic that took a painful toll on Iraq, whose healthcare has been devastated by decades of negligence.

Protests and the Exploitation of Brutality

On 1 October 2019, two weeks after my arrival, a group of Iraqi youth demonstrated demanding employment opportunities and protesting the inequality between the privileged political parties and the rest of the population. This routine popular eruption has always been contained by government announcements of new jobs in the oversaturated public sector or faded away after the demonstrators made their voice heard. But this time it was dramatically different. The protestors were met with disproportionate force that led to dozens of deaths and many injuries among the demonstrators, who in turn violently attacked the Iraqi security forces. The next ten days witnessed widespread violence and more killings and injuries as the country moved steadily toward the abyss. All this was happening in the midst of complete absence of political leadership. Prime Minister Adil Abdul-Mahdi did not address the nation until 4 October, and when he decided to do so, he delivered his address in the most inexplicable fashion – his speech was broadcast on Iraqi National Television well past mid-night and was quite uninspiring. But his government was saved by a 1,338 year old memory, as millions of Iraqis began preparing for the traditional walk toward Karbala to commemorate the martyrdom of Imam Hussain, the grandson of Prophet Mohammed.[1] The demonstrators suspended their protests and promised a strong return on 25 October to avoid a conflict between their activities and the religious pilgrimage.

The return of protests took the country on a political rollercoaster as the staggering violence led to hundreds of deaths and thousands of injuries. On 29 November 2019, Prime Minister Adil Abdul-Mahdi submitted his resignation citing the Friday Prayer sermon by Grand Ayatollah Sistani's Representative, "the hard conditions of the country and to allow for a better chance calm the situation and give the Council of Representatives (CoR) a chance to consider new options".[2] This was the first time an Iraqi government resigned since 2003. Encouraged by this accomplishment, the demonstrators stepped up their protests and, under their tremendous pressure, the Iraqi CoR began the process of introducing several reforms to address popular demands that fell on deaf ears for over fifteen years. Iraq was heading towards a game change before another exogenous development took precedence over the domestic power struggle. A rocket attack on Iraq's K1 military base near Kirkuk, which hosts US troops, caused the death of one American contractor and multiple injuries among other servicemen.[3] The US blamed

---

[1] This annual event attracts an estimated 15 million Iraqis who walk from their places of residence to Imam Husain's shrine in Karbala to commemorate his martyrdom in 681 A.D. They are normally joined by hundreds of thousands from other countries who travel to Iraq for the occasion, known as the *Arba'een* (the passing of forty days after the actual martyrdom anniversary). This annual event attracts an estimated 15 million Iraqis who walk from their places of residence to Imam Husain's shrine in Karbala to commemorate his martyrdom in 681 A.D. They are normally joined by hundreds of thousands from other countries who travel to Iraq for the occasion, known as the *Arba'een* (the passing of forty days after the actual martyrdom anniversary).

[2] A.J. Rubin and F. Hassan, "Iraqi Prime Minister Resigns in Deepening Political Crisis", *The New York Times*, 30 November 2019.

[3] E. McLaughlin and L. Martinez, "US civilian contractor killed, several troops

Kataib Hezbollah, an Iraqi paramilitary group linked to Iran, and retaliated on 29 December by conducting strikes against three of the group's bases in Iraq and two in Syria. The attacks resulted in 25 deaths and 51 injuries.[4] Kataib Hezbollah and other Popular Mobilization Forces (PMF) allied with them responded to this attack by besieging the US Embassy in Baghdad, a scene that reminded observers of the 1979 takeover of the US Embassy in Tehran.[5]

Prime Minister Adil Abdul-Mahdi used a combination of coercion and persuasion on the leaders of the siege and managed to secure their withdrawal from the US Embassy's vicinity. He promised to handle the security issues and ensure that US forces operate according to the mutual agreements and under the supervision of the Iraqi government, as a condition of their operating in Iraq. Abdul-Mahdi was notified about the 29 December US airstrikes on the Kataib, but no details were provided to him regarding the timing and target locations, which earned him harsh criticism from many Iraqis.

The last straw came in the form of a US airstrike near Baghdad International Airport that left a few Iraqis and Iranians dead, including Major General Qasem Soleimani, the commander of the Quds Force, a branch of the Iranian Islamic Revolutionary Guards Corps (IRGC), and Abu Mahdi al-Muhandis, the deputy chief of the PMF.[6] The former was on a visit to Iraq to meet Prime Minister Adil Abdul-Mahdi while the latter was receiving him at the airport. The attack triggered many uncomfortable questions about the nature of US-Iraqi relations and the status of the US forces that operate

---

injured in rocket attack on Iraqi military base", *ABC News*, 27 December 2019.

[4] US Attacks Iran-backed Militia Bases in Iraq and Syria", *BBC News*, 30 December 2019.

[5] F. Hassan, B. Hubbard, and A.J. Rubin, "Protesters Attack US Embassy in Iraq, Chanting 'Death to America'", *The New York Times*, 31 December 2019.

[6] The PMF, also known as the Popular Mobilization Units (PMU) or Popular Mobilization Committee (PMC), is an umbrella group composed of militias of varying sizes and political affiliations that are officially part of the Iraqi Security Forces.

on Iraqi soil and air space. The fact that they were conducted with no coordination with the Iraqi government and without Abdul-Mahdi's knowledge forced the Prime Minister to reverse his position on the presence of US troops. He went to the CoR and appealed to the legislature to pass a resolution mandating a complete withdrawal of US troops from Iraq.[7]

The Soleimani killing and its aftermath also had a direct effect on the demonstrators throughout Iraq, who for months had been calling for anti-corruption reforms and an end to foreign interference, especially Iran's influence. These demands were forced to take a back seat as pro-democracy protestors in Iraq came under overwhelming pressure to postpone their push for change. US-Iraq relations were brought to their lowest point in recent memory, and even the most vocal Iraqi supporters of the United States had to disappear from the scene.

Media attention immediately shifted from the Iraqi protesters to the more newsworthy rapid escalation in the US-Iran conflict, and once again, demands for political reform in Iraq were eclipsed by higher national priorities. Instead of replacing the corrupt election law and reforming the controversial High Elections Commission, the Iraqi CoR passed a highly consequential resolution calling on the government to expel all US troops from Iraq.

The Double Crisis:
Political Stalemate and the Oil Curse

Iraq is a rentier state, with 93% of its budget reliant on oil revenues. Like many oil producing countries, Iraq has limited control over production quantities and prices. Iraq started its 2020 revenues with oil prices hovering over US$60/barrel. With its level of production being around 4.5mbd, including oil used for domestic consumption, the country barely breaks even on salaries, mandatory financial obligations, and partial

---

[7] *Iraqi Parliament Calls for Troop Withdrawal What Next for the United States?*, Atlantic Council, 5 January 2020.

basic services. In the first quarter, Iraq produced an average of 4.6mbd,[8] as prices started to decline from US\$63.65/barrel in January to US\$55.66/barrel in February and US\$32.01/barrel in March.[9] The second quarter started with another dramatic price decrease to reach US\$18.38 in April and US\$29.38 in May, before it rose to US\$40.27 in June.[10] Meanwhile, Iraqi production went down to 4.7mbd in April and significantly decreased to 3.7mbd in May and June, setting the country into a deep financial crisis.[11]

The government of Adil Abdul-Mahdi, which turned into a caretaker status, took a hands-off attitude toward the country's staggering hardships as President Barham Salih and major political leaders in the CoR struggled to form a new government. Two candidates for Prime Minister were rejected before they got the chance to have a vote in the CoR and were forced to withdraw their names from the race to set the stage for National Intelligence Chief Mustafa al-Kadhimi to be confirmed as a compromise Prime Minister on 7 May 2020. The leaders who appointed Prime Minister al-Kadhimi gave him a mandate to focus on the following priorities: preparing for an early election, restoring Iraqi sovereignty and bringing all arms under state control, and leading Iraq through the economic crunch and Covid-19 crisis. He added to that the promise to conduct a swift and credible investigation into the waves of violence beginning in October 2019 and bring the culprits to justice, as well as fight corruption wherever it may be found.[12]

---

[8] Iraq Crude Oil Production, *Trading Economics*.

[9] "Numbers cited refer to average monthly Brent crude oil price", *Statista*, 20 July 2020.

[10] Ibid.

[11] Iraq Crude Oil Production…, cit.

[12] For a copy of the full program, see "NAS publishes the full text of the ministerial program of the government of Mustafa Al-Kadhimi", Baghdad, NAS.

The Impact of Covid-19 on
Government-Opposition Relations

From the beginning of the pandemic's outbreak, Iraq was identified as a very vulnerable state because of its fragile administrative system, depleted healthcare sector, and lack of economic and financial resources. To make matters worse, Iraq's closest neighbor, Iran, became the second epicenter of the Covid-19 pandemic after its country of origin, China. Iran has also been the main destination for the majority of Iraqis who travel abroad. Hundreds of thousands choose Iran for recreation and religious tourism, medical treatment, and business-related travel. A significantly larger number of Iranians in turn visit Iraq for religious tourism to the holy shrines in Karbala, Najaf, Baghdad, and Samarra, in addition to Iranian students who move back and forth between the two leading Shia seminaries in Najaf, Iraq and Qom, Iran. Many asymptomatic travelers returned to Iraq carrying the virus in the early days and spread it to their families and communities.

During the months of pandemic Iraq lost athletes, including three legendary football players, poets, artists, community leaders, and politicians. Many others were lucky to survive after contracting the disease. In a philosophical reaction to the pandemic, the Iraqi academic Dr. Hassan Nadhim posted to his Facebook page a note on the "four humiliations of human narcissism" at the hands of Copernicus, Darwin, Freud, and Covid-19.[13] On 26 June, a few weeks after he was confirmed as Iraq's Minister of Culture in Mustafa al-Kadhimi's government, Dr. Nadhim tested positive for Covid-19. After a few weeks of wrestling with the virus, he reflected on the battle he won:

> Both the virus and I were exhausted. Both of us witnessed metamorphoses. While the virus witnessed the metamorphoses of Covid and I witnessed the metamorphoses of Ovid, we reconsidered our own myths and symbols. We, both, went

---

[13] https://www.facebook.com/hassan.nadhcm.5/posts/10221738341957259

> through a kind of false tranquility, we rose against each other, we raged, rebelled, persisted, and felt desperate. I could hear it and feel it in me, Covid and Ovid. … But finally, after a few days, it fell asleep and was quiet ever since. The visible and invisible struggles have come to an end.[14]

In addition to impacting Iraqi culture, the pandemic had a significant effect on social movements in the country. In the weeks prior to the spread of Covid-19, Iraqi protesters began to re-group and recover the momentum they lost during the US-Iran escalation. Their goal was to force the CoR to enact several reform legislations that would change the electoral system, contain corruption, and end the monopoly of ruling political parties on employment, business contracts, and access to national and local decision making. Having already resigned, the government of Prime Minister Adil Abdul-Mahdi had nothing to lose from the success of the protest movement. But the political establishment was losing ground everyday as the pressure on them mounted from the streets of Baghdad and key provinces. When the Covid-19 pandemic became a public concern, the pressure started to fade away.[15] Large crowds disappeared from the streets and the televised suffering of Covid-19 patients convinced everyone that the government ban on large gatherings was justified, regardless of the political motivations behind it. Most of the protesters were content to retreat temporarily to preserve their lives, wait for the pandemic to recede, and return later to continue the fight. Meanwhile, political leaders reversed their positions on reform and appointed a government on straight partisan quota (*muhassassa*).[16]

It is unclear whether the pandemic will strengthen the political regime's control over the Iraqi society, or the opposite is more

---

[14] https://www.facebook.com/hassan.nadhem.5/posts/10222803088975269

[15] The first coronavirus case appeared in Iraq in February 2020. See: "Iraq takes new decisions to confront COVID-19 as infections reach 315,597", *Xinhuanet*, 19 September 2020.

[16] A.H. Cordesman, *Iraq is the Prize: A Warning About Iraq's Future Stability, Iran, and the Role of the United States*, Center for Strategic and International Studies (CSIS), 20 March 2020.

likely to happen. In the short term, the fear of infection by the deadly virus drove large crowds away from the streets and places of protest. The political elite have bought some valuable time and enjoyed a temporary relief from the political and security pressures. But, in the long term, it is more likely to empower the opposition as the economic and social consequences take their toll. Meanwhile, the government will use pandemic-related public health concerns as a pretext to impose extended curfew periods and other legal restrictions on public activities. Deploying such legal and security devices in a deceptive way may make it difficult to mobilize the necessary opposition forces in the short run, but this could be a double-edged sword and increase the gap between the government and the population. In this case, a heavy price will have to be paid in the coming elections. Political opposition may exploit what the pandemic exposed about the regime's shortcomings in preparing for and addressing the health crisis. However, whether or not they are exploited by the opposition, these vulnerabilities are destined to haunt the political regime as the long-term economic effects of the pandemic make their impact on several key sectors and aggravate the poor conditions of wide segments of Iraqi population.

Conclusion

For the past seventeen years, Iraq has been moving in a cyclical pattern of violence. Ethno-sectarian politics have prevailed over creative governance and divisive discourse has often paid off better than the message of unity and social cohesion. The state has maintained a rentier economy with more than 90% of the national budget drawn from the petroleum sector. Many sectors that made significant contributions to the Iraqi economy in the past were devastated by greedy influential politicians who made fortunes from monopolies on imports at the expense of national products.

The impact of rampant corruption on the Iraqi infrastructure has been felt throughout the country. Billions of US dollars were spent on electricity, roads, schools, and hospitals, but the reality on the ground does not match these expenditures. Until the 1980s, Iraq possessed one of the best healthcare systems in the entire region. This system crumbled slowly under the crippling sanctions that were imposed by the UN Security Council between 1990 and 2003. Although the post-2003 era opened a window of opportunity to restore the Iraqi healthcare industry, fraud, waste, and mismanagement left the country in hopeless conditions. Hospitals are completely depleted and run by incompetent cronies of the ruling political parties, while doctors are under-paid and unprotected. They are open to physical attacks by unruly mobs and threatened by tribal retaliation for actual or perceived malpractice.[17]

When the Covid-19 pandemic reached Iraq, this vulnerability presented the Iraqi people with the sobering reality of how broken their country really is. The country was paralyzed by a shortage of medicine, protective equipment, hospital beds, and medical staff. Furthermore, public health awareness and prevention measures were almost non-existent, because the country has not invested in this important tool of healthcare preparedness. A significantly large percentage of Iraqis remain under-educated or not educated at all.[18] Many preferred to follow religious guidance rather than medical instructions, and simple government guidelines such as observing social distancing and reducing unnecessary social and religious activities proved impossible to enforce. As for those who trusted these guidelines, they too found themselves obligated to violate them because of the devastating economic conditions. For too many Iraqis, staying home meant certain death by starvation, so they decided to take their chances with the virus, which after all had a killing rate of 3% or less.

---

[17] "Iraq doctors say vendettas threaten their lives as they save others", *France24*, 28 February 2019.
[18] "Country at a Glance - Iraq", Education Statistics, World Bank.

It was thought that the post-ISIS era would herald new challenges for Iraq.[19] That prediction began to materialize after a short-lived national euphoria: the triple crisis of protests, severe economic hardship, and Covid-19 will set the scene for a perfect storm if the Iraqi political leadership continue their reckless conduct.

---

[19] International Crisis Group, "Post-ISIS Iraq: A Gathering Storm", 26 October 2003.

5. Socio-Economic and Political Impact of Covid-19 on the GCC States

Gawdat Bahgat

For many years political analysts have argued that the rentier-economy and welfare-state model in the Gulf Cooperation Council (GCC) states (Bahrain, Kuwait, Oman, Qatar, Saudi Arabia and the United Arab Emirates) is un-sustainable.[1] For decades GCC governments have provided their citizens with education, health care, guaranteed employment, and many other public services and material benefits free, or almost free, of charge in return for political acquiescence, the so-called, "no taxation, no representation bargain".[2] At least since the early 2000s many scholars of the Gulf region have called on the states to re-negotiate the social contract, meaning imposing taxes and, in return, giving their citizens some political rights, including having a voice in how their governments are run.

This chapter argues that this call for re-writing the social contract is a valid and reasonable argument, but the time for its full implementation has not come yet. For several years the GCC states have imposed and collected taxes and their citizens have been granted some space to exercise a number of political rights. They are not one-man authoritarian regimes like Saddam Hussein's Iraq or Muammar Gaddafi's Libya, rather, most

---

[1] Gregory III Gause, *Oil Monarchies: Domestic and Security Challenges in the Arab Gulf States*, New York, Council on Foreign Relations, 1994.

[2] H. Beblawi and G. Luciani, *The Rentier State: Nation, State and Integration in the Arab World*, London and New York, Croom Helm, 1987.

political decisions are made by consensus between different tribal and societal leaders. Different formal and informal power centers participate in the decision-making process. The voice of public opinion and civil society is growing louder. Certainly, this cannot be solely attributed to the state's diminishing financial capabilities. Rather, the revolution in information technology and social media has contributed to the rise of citizens' participation in the political process and demand for transparency, accountability, and good governance.

However, these trends are modest; much more is still needed. For example, according to the latest report by Freedom House, only Kuwait is "partly free", while the other five GCC states are "not free".[3] Gulf rulers enjoy tremendous power and are not likely to give it up any time soon. Since March 2020, the Covid-19 pandemic has dealt a heavy blow to socio-economic activities in the GCC, like it has in the rest of the world. But, as this chapter will demonstrate, the GCC governments are better prepared to deal with these crises than most other countries. They are well-equipped to overcome any opposition to their rule by offering a combination of significant rewards and severe punishments. Furthermore, given the Gulf governments' substantive investments around the world and lucrative arms deals, their abuse of basic human rights is less scrutinized than the case in other countries.

The Dual Crises – Covid-19 and Collapse of Oil Prices

Since late 2010, the GCC states and the broader Middle East have been dealing with numerous political and security challenges created by the so-called Arab Spring. However, unlike some of their neighbors, the Gulf leaders have survived the political uprising. The most vulnerable state was Bahrain, given

---

[3] Freedom House, Freedom in the World 2020, "A Leaderless Struggle for Democracy".

its sectarian composition and the fact that it is not as rich as some of its neighbors. Still, Kuwait, Qatar, Saudi Arabia, and the UAE provided generous financial assistance to their less wealthy GCC member-states Bahrain and Oman. In addition to their ability to successfully manage the political storm at home, some of the GCC states have been involved in regional crises including civil wars in Syria, Libya, and Yemen and intense economic pressure in Egypt. These active regional roles have proved costly both politically and financially. It is not clear how much domestic support Gulf governments enjoy in their interventions in regional conflicts, but the international community has strongly condemned foreign intervention in Yemen and Libya. Furthermore, Gulf states' involvement in regional conflicts has added more restraints on their financial systems.

It was in the midst of these tensions that Covid-19 hit. The Gulf region, and indeed the entire world, was not prepared. The virus has triggered the deepest global recession since World War II. This is a crisis like no other and there is substantial uncertainty about its impact on people's lives and livelihoods. Much depends on the epidemiology of the virus, the effectiveness of containment measures and the development of therapeutics and vaccines, all of which are hard to predict.[4] In response, widespread policy measures have been implemented to help limit the spread of infection. These include the cancellation of large public events, restrictions on air travel, and the closure of schools and government offices. Recent relaxations to mitigation measures have been gradual. Large economic stimulus packages have been offered in the GCC states (and elsewhere). These packages have included measures on health spending, social assistance, and support to small businesses. Since the GCC central banks are pegged with the US dollar, they cut rates in tandem with emergency cuts by the US Federal Reserve.

---

[4] G. Gopinath, "The great lockdown: worst economic downturn since the great depression", IMFBlog, 14 April 2020.

The MENA oil exporting countries have been hit by two shocks simultaneously – Covid-19 and the oil price collapse. Stated differently, the severe socio-economic and political impact of the pandemic and global lockdown has been further aggravated by the huge decline of oil prices – the main source of income for all GCC states. True to its inherent nature, the price of oil has seen unprecedented volatility in the last decade during two main crises. The first occurred mid-2014; prices collapsed from more than US$100/barrel in early 2014 to around US$30/barrel in early 2016.[5] Prices partially recovered until their collapse in early 2020, following the global spread of Covid-19.

Since the dawn of the oil era, prices have been subject to a certain extent of volatility. But the depth of change in early 2020 was unprecedented. At the start of the year, one barrel of oil was sold for over US$60, but on 20 April, the price of West Texas Intermediary (WTI), the US benchmark for light crude, fell well into negative territory for the first time in history. Sellers had to pay customers to take unwanted oil – an unimaginable and untenable ask of the industry. Like any commodity, the price of oil reflects the balance between supply and demand. The drastic changes in daily social and economic activities around the world in response to the Covid-19 pandemic have pushed the global oil market out of balance. On the supply side, in March the members of the Organization of Petroleum Exporting Countries (OPEC) and other major producers, mainly Russia, were unable to extend a previous agreement signed to cut production a few years ago. This failure permitted a lift of all restrictions and major producers started competing for the market share. In early April, the global market was flooded with a substantial surplus. This excessive production prompted world leaders to renegotiate a new oil deal under which OPEC members and other producers agreed

---

[5] Shebabi, *Quantifying Dutch Disease Effects and Asymmetry in Economic Responses to Oil Price Volatility in Kuwait*, The Oxford Institute for Energy Studies, July 2020.

to cut production. This agreement was further endorsed by the world's largest economies through the G20.

On the demand side, daily global consumption fell by approximately 30 million barrels in early 2020. This significant collapse in consumption is likely to persist for some time in light of the ongoing global health crisis. Refineries are unwilling to turn oil into gasoline, diesel, and other products because so few people are commuting or taking airplane flights and international trade has slowed sharply. This combination of excessive production and substantial reduction in utilization has created a new challenge concerning global storage facilities for the abundance of oil the industry continues to pump out. In a nutshell, there is an enormous global surplus met with little demand, and possible storage venues are dwindling. Until the Covid-19 pandemic eases and economic growth returns, downward price pressure will continue.

The GCC States' Response to the Two-Fold Crisis

The Gulf Arab states, like the rest of the world, were overwhelmed with the rapid and devastating spread of Covid-19, which, among other things, contributed to the collapse of oil prices. Since March 2020, they have focused their efforts on mitigating the short term and long term impacts of these two crises. A key challenge is that strategies for addressing both must be adopted in an environment of very high uncertainty. There is a great deal of uncertainty regarding if and when the virus will be contained and subsequently on the shape and speed of national, regional, and global economic recovery. This means that Covid-19 containment is strongly connected to the rise in oil demand. In other words, the health crisis and the oil price collapse overlap with one another.

Confronted with this two-fold crisis, the GCC governments, like other governments around the world, imposed lockdowns, closed schools and mosques, banned gatherings and even scaled down the pilgrimage/*hajj*. They also laid off millions of foreign laborers. Accurate figures on their financial losses are not yet available, but in April 2020 the International Monetary Fund (IMF) projected that growth in the MENA region will contract by more than 4% and in the GCC states by 2.7% in 2020, and the current account will shift from a surplus of 5.6% of GDP in 2019 to a deficit of 3.1% of GDP in 2020. Three months into the Covid-19 crisis, the IMF revised the projection to a larger growth decline of 4.7%.[6] This more pessimistic outlook is due to the sharp decline in oil prices and disruptions in trade and tourism triggered by the pandemic. In the coming few years, governments will be forced to cut spending, raise borrowing, and delay or halve government investments. Despite this gloomy short-term economic outlook, the sky is not falling. The medium to long term outlook looks bright. Both the IMF and the World Bank project that economic growth will accelerate in 2021. The real GDP rate (adjusted for inflation) in all six states will grow:[7]

	Real GDP Growth	
	2020	**2021**
Bahrain	-3.6	3.0
Kuwait	-1.1	3.4
Oman	-2.8	3.0
Qatar	-4.3	5.0
Saudi Arabia	-2.3	2.9
UAE	-3.5	3.3

World Bank analysts echo similar sentiments. They project that the GCC economies will rebound from -4.1% in 2020 to 2.2% in 2021. This optimistic projection is based on several assumptions, including that: the pandemic subsides, investment recovers, foreign investment restrictions relax, regulatory

---

[6] International Monetary Fund, *Regional Economic Outlook: Middle East and Central Asia*, 2020 Update, 13 July 2020.
[7] Ibid.

environments improve and diversification programs continue.[8]
Furthermore, long ago, the GCC states (and other countries)
created sovereign wealth funds (SWFs), also known as oil
funds.[9] These include the Abu Dhabi Investment Authority
(1976), Kuwait Investment Authority (1953), Qatar Investment
Authority (2005) and the Saudi Public Investment Fund
(1971). Over the last few decades, these funds have accumulated
substantial financial assets. In early 2020, the Sovereign Wealth
Funds Institute provided the following estimates:[10]

Abu Dhabi Investment Authority (ADIA)	US$580 billion
Emirates Investment Authority (EIA)	US$45 billion
Kuwait Investment Authority (KIA)	US$239 billion
Investment Corporation of Dubai (ICD)	US$534 billion
Mubadala Investment Company	US$232 billion
Bahrain Mumtalakat Holding Company	US$19 billion
Public Investment Fund	US$360 billion
Qatar Investment Authority (QIA)	US$295 billion
Sharjah Asset Management	US$793 million

These huge financial assets mean that despite the heavy blow
Covid-19 has dealt to the GCC's economies, the global system,
and oil prices, the rentier state is not about to collapse. As in
previous crises, the GCC governments are likely to utilize some
of their financial reserves in these SWFs to stimulate their
economies, buy off their opponents and keep the majority of
their citizens happy. The SWFs provide the GCC states with
large financial cushions and serve as buffers against short-term
economic downturn and political instability. These buffers are
depleting, but they remain adequate for most GCC states.

[8] World Bank Group, *Global Economic Prospects*, June 2020.
[9] Xu Yi-chong and G. Bahgat, *The political economy of sovereign wealth funds*, London,
Palgrave Macmillan, 2010.
[10] Sovereign Wealth Fund Institute (SWFI), *List of 25 sovereign wealth fund profiles
in Middle East*.

Political Opposition

There is no doubt that the GCC states were not prepared to address the enormous health challenges triggered by Covid-19. Adding fuel to the fire, the outbreak of Covid-19 and the wide-ranging measures introduced to slow its advance have precipitated an unprecedented collapse in oil demand, a surge in oil inventories and, in March 2020, the steepest one-month decline in oil prices on record.

It is important to neither overestimate nor underestimate the socio-economic and political impact of this two-fold crisis. Compared with other regional powers, certainly, the GCC states collectively have not handled the crisis as well as Jordan has, but they have done much better than neighboring Iran. Figures from World Health Organization and Johns Hopkins University compare the GCC states' Covid-19 response to that of both Jordan and Iran as of early August 2020:

Country	Infected cases	Deaths[11]	Deaths/100k pop[12]
Bahrain	43,307	161	10.13%
Kuwait	70,727	471	11.28%
Oman	81,067	502	10.39%
Qatar	112,383	180	6.47%
Saudi Arabia	285,793	3,093	9.18%
UAE	62,061	356	3.70%
Jordan	1,237	11	0.11%
Iran	322,567	18,152	22.17%

In addition to these efforts to contain the virus, the GCC governments, like some other regimes, have taken advantage of the emerging uncertainty to further expand their strict

---

[11] World Health Organization, "WHO Coronavirus Disease (Covid-19) Dashboard", 2020.

[12] Johns Hopkins University & Medicine, Coronavirus resource Center, Mortality Analyses, 2020.

restrictions on civil society and any potential political opposition. Although declaring a state of emergency is not inherently illegal, it is evident that a number of governments around the world are using this constitutional tool to severely restrict fundamental freedoms, such as freedom of information, expression, assembly and association. In reality, many measures that were imposed with the pretext of combatting the pandemic are in fact being used as an excuse to repress government opposition.

Furthermore, there has been an increase in the use of surveillance technology as a means to track the spread of the virus. On one hand, this practice has an advantage in that people who have come into contact with an infected person are immediately informed so that they can be tested and remain in self-quarantine. On the other hand, this practice can, and indeed has been used to, encroach on the privacy of citizens as authorities are able to monitor political opponents and their movements. This means that Covid-19 has become both a major public health threat and, simultaneously, could lead to severe restrictions on individuals' privacy and freedom of movement.[13]

In 2020, the UAE enacted a temporary law that allows the authorities to access individuals' WhatsApp calls and conversations, as well as their Skype and Google accounts. In addition, people residing in the country must complete an online form explaining a valid reason for their trip when leaving their homes. This form should be presented to the authorities if questioned on the street. The law gives the government access to the individuals' biometric identifications, phone numbers, and car license plate numbers. The tracking technology has been used to identify people who violate imposed social distancing measures as well as to track down individuals who allegedly spread "false information".[14]

---

[13] M. Hedges, "Gulf States Use Coronavirus Threat to Tighten Authoritarian Controls and Surveillance", *The conversation*, 21 April 2020.
[14] A. Admin, *Covid-19: How the Pandemic Used by GCC Governments to Double Down on Human Rights Violations*, Americans for Democracy & Human Rights in Bahrain,

Conclusion

It is too early to provide an accurate assessment of the medium and long term impact of the Covid-19 crisis on the socio-economic and political environment in the GCC states. The analysis in this chapter identifies three trends. First, governments in the Gulf and around the world are playing a bigger role in the economy to combat the pandemic and provide economic lifelines to peoples and firms. This expanded role is crucial but it also increases opportunities for corruption. To help ensure the money and measures are helping the people who need it most, governments need timely and transparent reporting, ex-post audits and accountability procedures, and close cooperation with civil society and the private sector. As public finances worsen, countries need to prevent the loss of funds caused by corruption in public spending.[15]

Second, the GCC governments have responded to the pandemic fallout by introducing more prohibitive immigration policies. An unspecified number of foreign workers had been sent back to their home countries. This deportation of tens of thousands of migrant workers is certain to have significant impact in both their countries of origin and in the Gulf states. For decades, human rights organizations have been monitoring the conditions of foreign workers in the Gulf states closely and have expressed concerns about their social welfare. Due to Covid-19, the unhygienic conditions of the overcrowded labor camps have further deteriorated. These include lack of access to clean running water and restricted access to basic medical care. Furthermore, living conditions and crowded camps make social distancing out of the question. It is not clear whether these foreign workers will be allowed to go back to the Gulf states when the virus is contained. Some of these states with small population (i.e. Kuwait, Qatar, United Arab Emirates)

---

1 June 2020.
[15] V. Gaspar, M. Muhleisen, and R. Weeks-Brown, "Corruption and Covid-19", IMFBlog, 28 July 2020.

cannot maintain their economic prosperity and their way of life without a large number of expatriates.

Thirds, despite the two-fold crisis due to the collapse of oil prices and Covid-19, it is important to emphasize that none of the GCC governments has experienced any serious political challenge. There is no well-organized, grass roots opposition. There are at least two reasons for this lack or weakness of such opposition. First, GCC states are generally among the richest countries in the world. They hold massive oil and natural gas reserves and over the years have accumulated substantial wealth. They use their financial muscles to brutally punish opponents and reward supporters. Second, given their lucrative investments around the world, Gulf states are under very little, if any, international pressure to introduce political reform and any real measures of transparency, freedom, and accountability.

Against this background, Gulf citizens who are not satisfied with how their governments have responded to the financial and health crises have turned to social media to air their grievances and/or have left their countries for the United States, Canada, or Europe. Chats on social media provide very modest criticism of official policies. Despite talk of political reforms, Gulf governments have strongly and brutally responded to any criticism of their policies. Their tactics include stripping opponents of their citizenships, long-term imprisonment, and even execution. For critics residing in the West, some GCC states have forced their families to pressure the dissenting relatives into silence, disown and discredit them, and denounce their actions. Families that fail to comply face travel bans, social isolation, job loss, and even incarceration.[16]

To sum up, despite the severity of the financial crisis, triggered partly by Covid-19 and the overwhelming rate of infection, there are no signs of any serious political opposition in any of the Gulf states. In Oman, Sultan Qaboos bin Said died on 10

---

[16] O. Salem, "Arab Dictators Are Learning to Love Collective Punishment", *Foreign Policy*, 4 August 2020.

January 2020 and was succeeded by his cousin Haitham bin Tariq in an ordinary fashion. The Emir of Kuwait Sabah al-Ahmad al-Jaber al-Sabah died on 29 September 2020, at 91 years old, and was succeeded by Nawaf al-Ahmad Al-Jaber Al-Sabah, who is 83 years old. The King of Saudi Arabia Salman bin Abdulaziz al-Saud is 84 years old. His son, Crown Prince Mohammad bin Salman has been consolidating his power since 2015. A close examination of the GCC states' responses to the Coronavirus crisis shows that there is mild criticism, but no well-organized dissent movements. If there will be any change, it is more likely to come from the top rather than the bottom. The information-technology revolution and the fact that the great majority of Gulf citizens are enjoying access to un-censored news and information suggest that a popular change might take place, but it is likely to take some time.

6. Iran: Access to Justice

Nadereh Chamlou

President Hassan Rouhani inaugurated the academic year amidst extensive uncertainty about the safety of students and teachers going back to classrooms, given that many regions in Iran had become again Covid-19 hotspots. But unlike previous years when the President rang in the new academic year with an in-person visit to a Tehran school, he did so this time via video.[1] Days earlier, a photo of Ayatollah Khamenei was released showing him sitting alone, in a big mosque, weeping during a private sermon in remembrance of Ashura.[2] [3] It was meant to be a message of devotion and that the day must be remembered no matter what. Instead the two images of the physically and socially distanced leaders reinforced the notion of an ever-widening gap between the aging rulers and the people.

Covid-19 has exposed every country's dysfunctions, vulnerabilities, and fault lines. Granted, the whole world was caught off guard and there was little knowledge about the nature of this new virus. Rich and poor nations all struggled, made mistakes and miscalculations. Nevertheless, some countries fared better. For instance, South Korea was initially the worst hit country outside China, but it acted vigorously

[1] "Iran | Rouhani Launches the Start of New School Year in a Video Conference Ceremony", *UNews*, 5 September 2020.

[2] "Leader Commemorates Ashura, Respects Coronavirus Health Protocols", *Al-Manar TV Lebanon*, 27 August 2020.

[3] "What Is Ashura?", *BBC News*, 6 December 2011, https://www.bbc.com/news/world-middle-east-16047713.

and less than 400 have died so far.[4] Vietnam is another case with just over a thousand cases and only 35 deaths at the time of this writing.[5] Interestingly, it is widely acknowledged that governments headed by women have done better, such as Germany, New Zealand, Taiwan, Iceland (among more).[6] [7] Among the countries that have paid a heavy price in terms of lives and livelihoods, there is Iran. By the end of September 2020, the Johns Hopkins Coronavirus Resource Center had placed Iran second in terms of observed case fatality ratio, and over 25,000 lives have been lost.[8]

Iran became one of the earliest hot spots after Wuhan.[9] Between December 2019 and January 2020 doctors in Qom, one of the religious epicenters in Iran, reported increasing numbers of patients afflicted with a strange respiratory illness. Authorities ignored the warnings because high turnouts were necessary for important occasions.[10] They were to signal the legitimacy of the regime – much like President Donald Trump's campaign rallies in the United States. Among them were the multi-city funeral processions for Qasem Soleimani (the Revolutionary Guard leader who was assassinated by US forces in Iraq on 3 January), the ten-day celebration of the 41st anniversary of the Islamic Republic in early February, and the 21 February parliamentary election.[11] These became

[4] "Worldometer - Real Time World Statistics", *Worldometer.*

[5] Ibid.

[6] A. Taub, "Why Are Women-Led Nations Doing Better with Covid-19?", *The New York Times*, 13 August 2020.

[7] T. Liji, "Covid-19 Outcomes Better in Countries with Female Leaders", *News-Medical.net*, 17 July 2020.

[8] Johns Hopkins University & Medicine, Coronavirus resource Center, Mortality Analyses, 2020.

[9] M. Behravesh, "The Untold Story of How Iran Botched the Coronavirus Pandemic", *Foreign Policy*, 24 March 2020.

[10] "Elections, Ties with China Shaped Iran's Coronavirus Response", *Reuters*, 2 April 2020.

[11] BBC Persian, مستند ایران، کرونا و روایت چند زندگی YouTube Video, 27:24, 17 September 2020.

super-spreader occasions. In addition, since the virus originated in China, Iran feared disrupting its economic ties, since Beijing became Iran's lifeline and most important partner in the wake of the breakdown of the nuclear deal. Qom in particular is home to a high concentration of Chinese people, with nearly 700 Chinese clerical students in the Qom Seminary.[12] China is also constructing a US$2.7 billion high-speed train route and a solar power plant near Qom.[13]

Even until mid-March, the official media downplayed the severity of the virus.[14] But with rising death tolls, the regime swallowed the bitter pill and declared a lock-down. The Iranian people complied even though the lockdown coincided with Norouz, the Iranian new year, which is a time for family visits and travel. Naturally, the tourist industry and the hospitality sector were heavily hit.

Despite the fact that even Saudi Arabia had suspended Hajj, the Muslim calendar's most important event, objection to closures of religious sites inside Iran came predominantly from prominent clergy.[15] [16] But, for now, the fist-clenching "Death to America", and "Death to Israel" ritual and the Friday prayers have been suspended, and religious sites operate below capacity. Nevertheless, a cantankerous debate arose about whether or not to observe Ashura when Covid-19 was ravaging cities again.[17] Ultimately, the government was pressured to move forward with commemorations, though with guidelines – such as

---

[12] Elections, ties with China shaped Iran's coronavirus response", *Reuters*, 2 April 2020.

[13] J. Gambrell, "'Virus at Iran's gates': How Tehran failed to stop outbreak", *AP News*, 17 March 2020.

[14] Koocheh, نویزیولت یاورپ یب یرجم زومآ تربع ناتساد YouTube Video, 17:12, 24 March 2020.

[15] J. Spyer, "Mullahs & Covid-19: Iran's Failing Response Reflects Regime's Priorities", *The Jerusalem Post*, 20 March 2020.

[16] "Saudi Tells Muslims to Wait on Hajj Plans amid Coronavirus Crisis", *Al Jazeera*, 31 March 2020.

[17] G. Esfandiari, "To Weep or Not To Weep: Iran Debates Holding Muharram During Pandemic", *RadioFreeEurope/RadioLiberty*, 3 August 2020.

physical-distanced, low-occupancy, open-air, mask-required events. For the fearful believers, even virtual processions and a Muharram video game were offered.[18]

But are Iranians really such faithful devotees to prioritize piety over public health? The data do not suggest so.

The Missing Shia

In 2020, a representatively weighted survey of a sample of around 40,000 Iranians over 19 years old was carried out by Gamaan Center of the University of Tilburg in The Netherlands.[19] [20] It shed light on an astonishing speed of secularization within Iran. In a country that is officially over 90% Shia Muslim, and where the dogma has been expounded for the past forty two years in everyday life, only 32% were willing to label their identity as Shia.

So, how does the rest of the population self-identify in terms of belief? (see below) According to Gamaan "around 5% said they were Sunni Muslim and 3% Sufi Muslim. Another 9% said they were atheists, along with 7% who preferred the label of spirituality. Among the other selected religions, 8% said they were Zoroastrians – which is more correct to be interpreted as a reflection of Persian nationalism, and a desire for an alternative to Islam, rather than strict adherence to the Zoroastrian faith. Around 0.5% said they were Christian and 0.6% as Jewish and Baha'is combined".[21] More than 60% of those raised in conservative families said that they no longer pray or fast, which is in line with the findings of a state-backed official

---

[18] F. Fassihi, Twitter post, 29 August 2020, 11:54 a.m., https://twitter.com/farnazfassihi/status/1299752340342419457.

[19] GAMAAN, "Secularization and Religious Diversity in Iran 2020", YouTube Video, 17:37, 7 September 2020.

[20] GAMAAN in English, GAMAAN, The Group for Analyzing and Measuring Attitudes in IRAN, 7 August 2018.

[21] P. Abdolmohammadi, *The Revival of Nationalism and Secularism in Modern Iran*, LSE Middle East Centre, 2015.

poll.[22] Interestingly, a comprehensive survey conducted in 1975 during the secular rule of the Shah found that over 80% of those surveyed said they prayed and fasted regularly.[23] Hence, despite the Islamic Republic's every effort to proselytize Shia Islam, the flight from religiosity has been formidable.

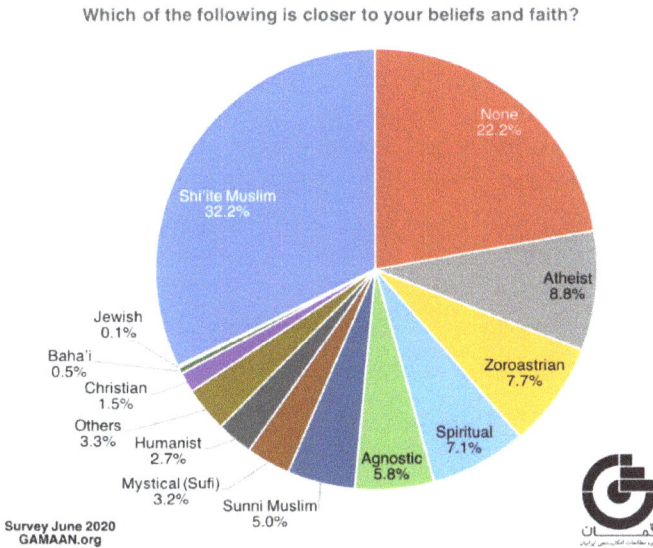

Which of the following is closer to your beliefs and faith?

Shi'ite Muslim 32.2%
None 22.2%
Atheist 8.8%
Zoroastrian 7.7%
Spiritual 7.1%
Agnostic 5.8%
Sunni Muslim 5.0%
Mystical (Sufi) 3.2%
Humanist 2.7%
Others 3.3%
Christian 1.5%
Baha'i 0.5%
Jewish 0.1%

Survey June 2020
GAMAAN.org

Source: GAMAAN, 2020 [24]

Based on these new findings, how strong could the support be for the regime's core ideology of "velayat-e faqih"?[25] Since it is a wholly Shia concept, we could assume that its followers must be among the Shia. But not every Shia would be in line with this doctrine. Is it safe to say that the supporters of the regime

[22] Ibid.

[23] A. Assadi and M.L. Vidale, "SURVEY OF SOCIAL ATTITUDES IN IRAN," *International Review of Modern Sociology*, vol. 10, no. 1, 1980, pp. 65-84.

[24] گَمان - گروه مطالعات افکارسنجی ایرانیان, (GAMAAN – The Group for Analyzing and Measuring Attitudes in IRAN), https://gamaan.org/

[25] K. Aarabi, *What Is Velayat-e Faqih?*, Institute for Global Change, 20 March 2019.

would amount to a fraction of the 32% self-identified Shia?

What have been the causes of this erosion of faith among a vast segment of the Shia population, so much so that it wants to disassociate itself from such identity? Much has been said and written about attributing the growing dissatisfaction of Iranians to the dire economic crisis that has led to a rise in income inequality, poverty, and unemployment. This article will not address these. Instead, it argues that the growing disconnect has also to do with (a) the expectations of an increasingly young, educated, urbanized post-revolution generation, and (b) the perception and experience of a population with a steadily worsening rule of law and unequal access to justice. Unlike economic conditions that may be influenced by external factors, such as sanctions or global economic shocks, the dimensions discussed below are shaped predominantly by internal dynamics, policies, and institutions.

Changing Demographics

The secularization is strongest among the younger age cohorts. Two out of three Iranians were born after the 1979 Revolution, resulting in a median age of 32 years.[26] With the sharply declining birth rates since the late 1980s, this generation was raised in smaller nuclear families, which are generally less prone to patriarchy and less conservative.[27] A second trend has been rapid urbanization. In 1979, two-thirds of Iran's 32 million population were rural; today, three-fourths of its 84 million are urban. Urbanization causes profound social transformation, such as openness and exposure to ideas and choices. This pattern can be observed in nearly all countries, as was witnessed in the US 2020 elections where urban areas voted predominantly for the Democrats while rural America was conservative and Republican.

---

[26] "Countries in the World by population (2020)", Worldometer.
[27] N. Chamlou, "Is Patriarchy on the Rise?", *World Bank Blogs*, 19 April 2012.

IRAN

2020 Population: 83,992,953

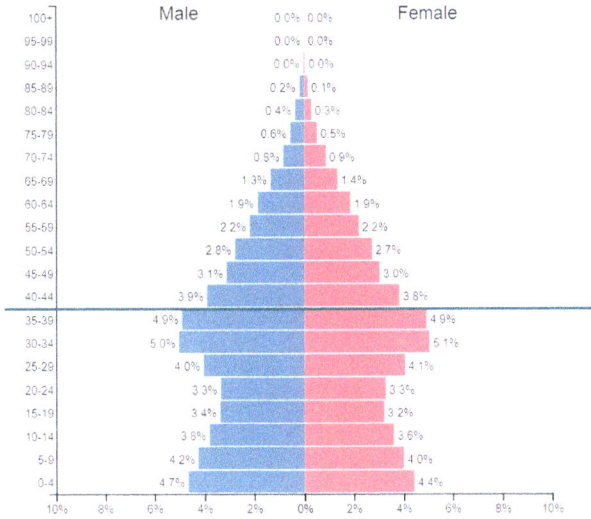

	Male			Female
100+		0.0%	0.0%	
95-99		0.0%	0.0%	
90-94		0.0%	0.0%	
85-89		0.2%	0.1%	
80-84		0.4%	0.3%	
75-79		0.6%	0.5%	
70-74		0.8%	0.9%	
65-69		1.3%	1.4%	
60-64		1.9%	1.9%	
55-59		2.2%	2.2%	
50-54		2.8%	2.7%	
45-49		3.1%	3.0%	
40-44		3.9%	3.8%	
35-39		4.9%	4.9%	
30-34		5.0%	5.1%	
25-29		4.0%	4.1%	
20-24		3.3%	3.3%	
15-19		3.4%	3.2%	
10-14		3.8%	3.6%	
5-9		4.2%	4.0%	
0-4		4.7%	4.4%	

■ Rural ■ Urban

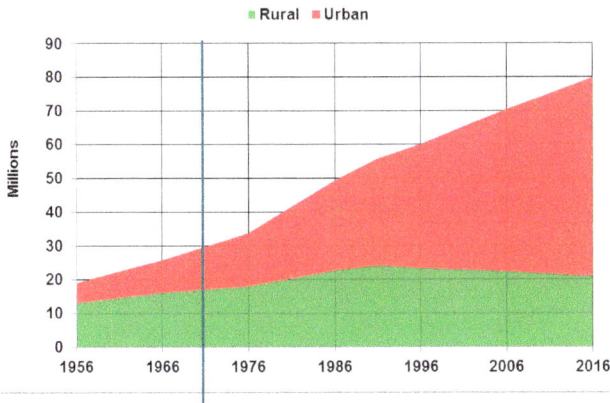

Source: Population Pyramids of the World from 1950 to 2100, PopulationPyramid.net

Capacity

Know-how

Deployment

Development

Iran, Islamic Rep. score

average score

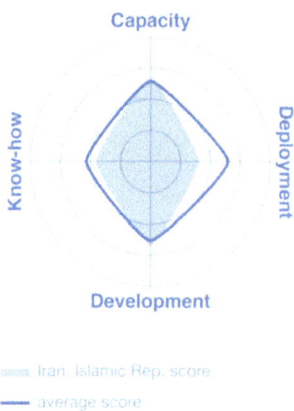

The third factor behind Iran's secularization trend is the expansion of education. The World Economic Forum's (WEF) Human Capital Report 2017 illustrates Iran's overall endowment (see figure).[28] While Iran ranks around global averages in terms of *capacity* (76th) and *development* (54th), it falls short in the categories of *know-how* (101st) and *deployment* (128th), the latter lowering the overall ratings to 104th among 130 countries. WEF defines *capacity* as a measure of formal educational attainment of the entire population, including the older age cohorts where literacy may have been low. *Deployment* measures the ability of the working age population to actually participate in the economy; it is depressed because of the low economic participation rate of women due to a host of legal and social impediments, as well as the high unemployment and underemployment in the economy that impacts the youth and first time job seekers. The *know-how* variable captures skill diversity and breadth of fields offered to recent university graduates. The *development* index is high, which is good news, and captures the formal education of the future workforce – a generation that is tech-savvy despite limitations and restrictions it has faced.[29] Indeed, Iranians are as connected as their peers globally. According to Gamaan, "levels of internet penetration in Iran are comparable to those in Italy, with some 60 million users, a number that grows steadily, and about 70% of adults subscribe to at least one social media platform."

---

[28] "The Global Human Capital Report 2017", World Economic Forum, 2017.
[29] A. Arouzi and D. De Luce, "Iranians Stay Connected on Social Media despite Regime Restrictions", *NBC News*, 24 August 2019.

The Covid-19 lockdown may have two long-term positive impacts: first, it pushed more and more citizens to become internet literate since nearly all goods and services are now obtained online. The government had to expand access, increase bandwidth, and loosen restrictions. This also afforded people to expand their online social networks during the time of physical distancing. Second, the absence of daily teachings of conservative government-required doctrines in schools opened the space for reinforcing intra-family values, introspections, and discussions, which are increasingly secular. Also, men had to take on some household duties and the care of children and the elderly. This made them more sensitive to the importance of sharing the burden and represents a gamechanger in terms of social norms and eroding deep-rooted notions of masculinity, as ongoing studies in several countries demonstrate.

Outcry about Recent Judicial Cases

As the United States was embroiled in demonstrations and riots in response to the systemic killing and oppression of Black people by police, there has been a global soul-searching around unequal application of the law and discrimination in access to justice for large groups of citizens. In Iran, too, there has been an ever-active movement for justice and fairness. In 2020, Iranians witnessed a new series of jaw-dropping cases. These include several political executions, a string of honor killings, and numerous high-profile cases of corruption and embezzlement.

Political executions

On September 12, the world woke up to the shocking news of the execution of Navid Afkari, a champion wrestler sentenced in relation to the presumed killing of an Iranian official.[30] The

---

[30] A. Moshtaghian, R. Mostaghim and I. Kottasova, "Navid Afkari Executed in

execution was despite a wide-ranging international plea by the public, leading sports entities, and UN agencies to halt the sentence, particularly since there was much unexplained, and the proof of guilt was based on a confession under torture. It is still not clear why there was a rush to execution. Weeks earlier another prisoner was executed even though he maintained his innocence, despite the harshest "interrogation techniques". Within days, an international public plea – #Don't_Execute – went viral when Iran's Supreme Court confirmed death sentences against three more young men (Amirhossein Moradi, Saeed Tamjidi and Mohammad Rajabi) on charges of taking part in arson and vandalism during the 2019 protests in response to the sudden threefold increase in fuel prices.[31] These protests were the worst the regime had experienced since the 1979 revolution.[32] Experts say social media has shed light on such executions, but that the regime may use these harsh punishments as a deterrent against future riots.

Violence against women and honor killings

The harshness of the inequality highlighted above pales in comparison to that seen in cases of violence against women and honor killings. In June alone, the public learnt of at least six chillingly documented cases in Abadan, Kerman, Kurdistan, and elsewhere.[33] [34] [35] In one case, a 14-year-old girl – Romina Ashrafi – was decapitated by her father with a sickle while

---

Iran despite International Campaign", *CNN,* 13 September 2020.
[31] S. Williams, "Don't Execute: Viral Campaign to Stop Iran Protester Hangings", *Digital Journal,* 14 August 2020.
[32] F. Fassihi and R. Gladstone, "With Brutal Crackdown, Iran Is Convulsed by Worst Unrest in 40 Years", *The New York Times,* 3 December 2019.
[33] "Iran's Police Confirmed the Fourth Case of Honor Killing in Less than a Month", *Iran International,* 19 June 2020.
[34] A. Cachia, "Iran Rocked by 'Honour Killing' as Man Kills Daughter with Iron Bar", *Daily Mail Online,* 18 June 2020.
[35] H. McKay, "From Poisonings to Beheadings, 'honor Killings' in Iran Gets a Fresh Spotlight with Social Media", *Fox News,* 26 June 2020.

sleeping.[36] To escape a life of domestic violence and threats by her father to kill her, she had eloped, but was returned home despite her pleas to the judge that her life would be in danger. Prior to the killing, Romina's father consulted with legal counsel about the kind of punishment he could expect by taking his daughter's life. Sharia law requires "an eye for an eye" and makes murder punishable by death – *qisas*. If a man kills another man, *qisas* will rule. But there are two exceptions. The first is an exemption in the penal code where a father's or paternal grandfather's killing a child is not a capital crime (this is not the case for a mother or anyone on the maternal side). The second is the killing of a woman by a man. Since a woman's *dieh* – blood money – is half of a man's, the killer can also avoid the death penalty. With little at stake, Romina's father beheaded her. Despite the act's horrific and premeditated nature, Romina's father was sentenced to a mere nine years.[37]

Iran is not the only country with honor killings; these happen even in the United States and Europe. The UN estimates around 5,000 women and girls become victims each year. The high-profile cases in Iran shed light on the prevalence of such crimes, which account for around 20% of all homicides. Statistics are difficult to obtain but are estimated around an average of 350-450 each year. In other words, every day at least one woman is killed at the hands of relatives, usually male. Still, experts suspect under-reporting. Amnesty International states that laws either do not recognize honor killings as a crime or the punishment is inadequate.[38]

A bill aimed at protecting women and girls against violence has been slow-walked for eight years in the Parliament, or *Majlis*, and other corridors of power. In 2014, several young

---

[36] B. Chakraborty, "Iranian Man Accused of Beheading 14-Year-Old Daughter in Honor Killing Arrested", *Fox News*, 28 May 2020.
[37] P. Wintour, "Outcry in Iran at Nine-Year Sentence for Man Who Beheaded Daughter", *The Guardian*, 28 August 2020.
[38] "The Horror of 'Honor Killings', Even in US", *Amnesty International USA*, 10 April 2012.

women in Isfahan were victims of acid attacks and were severely disfigured. The offenders have still not been found; it was rumored that the assault was instigated by a clerical hardliner. Victims were told in 2018 that the case had closed.[39] By contrast, the very same authorities were able to swiftly find the six youngsters who recorded a video of themselves dancing to Pharrell Williams' "Happy" from the roof top of their homes and posted it on social media.[40] They were sentenced to one year in prison and 91 lashes. But the cruelty in Romina's case set off public outcry that the law fails to protect women and children. In response, President Rouhani asked Parliament to expedite the bill.[41] Criminalizing such violence would be a first step to changing social norms.

Corruption in high places

While the above themes are shocking and heart-wrenching, a third category of court cases shook the Iranian public over the summer of 2020. They revealed the depth and breadth of yet another series of systemic corruption at the highest levels. Embezzlements in the banking sector or industry surface from time to time, some culprits flee abroad; some are jailed or even executed. This time, the spotlight is on the judiciary.[42] It is widely believed that many judges are corrupt, but the scale of the systemic corruption was astounding. Some 63 private bank accounts were discovered belonging to former judiciary chief Sadegh Amoli Larijani, funded largely from bail monies and other judicial fines and fees. "It was revealed that Larijani earned

---

[39] M. Lipin, "Iranian Acid Attack Victim Pursues Legal Fight Despite Claim 'Case Closed'", *Voice of America*, 20 July 2018.
[40] "Iran: Happy Video Dancers Sentenced to 91 Lashes and Jail", *BBC News*, 19 September 2014.
[41] F. Fassihi, "A Daughter Is Beheaded, and Iran Asks If Women Have a Right to Safety", *The New York Times*, 2 July 2020.
[42] P. Stone, "The Systematic Corruption in Iran's Judiciary", *Iran Focus*, 15 June 2020.

over US$66.5 million from these accounts' profits annually"[43] followed by reports that the proceeds were used for personal matters. But this was the tip of the iceberg; an elaborate bribery network was discovered to intervene in judicial cases. Some judges were given prime property, for instance, as a sign of "friendship", as one of the main culprits, the former executive deputy to Larijani, declared. He went on trial and was sentenced to 31 years in prison. Another judge implicated in the case for a half million Euro "gift" fled abroad and was later found dead in his hotel lobby in Romania under suspicious circumstances, reportedly a suicide.[44]

A few days later, on official TV, the Head of the Foundation for the Dispossessed (Bonyad Mostazafin), uttered some startling revelations. After the revolution, the Foundation routinely expropriated assets and property of pre-revolutionary industrialists and officials and used the vast proceeds to support the poor. He reported that some of the prime properties in upscale locations had been in use by regime insiders for personal purposes at little or no cost. Since some of those mentioned in his report were close to the Supreme Leader, he backtracked and downplayed his earlier statements by saying that they had gotten the permission of Ayatollah Khamenei to do so.[45] Nonetheless, the public came away with the impression that high officials were privy to excessive perks and benefits.

History of Iranian Legal System

Until the early XX century, Iran had no written or codified laws. The justice system consisted of a traditional Islamic practice in which each religious judge applied his own interpretation of

---

[43] Ibid.

[44] "Iranian Judge in Romania Died of Impact from Fall, Autopsy Says", *Reuters*, 23 June 2020.

[45] Koocheh, "پرویز فتاح حاتم یاهزرم طلغ مدرک ار اج هب اج درک" ("Parviz Fattah moved the wrong borders"), YouTube Video, 19:51, 19 August 2020.

the Shari'a. The primary demands of Iranian Constitutionalists were a bill of rights and the establishment of an "Edalatkhaneh" ("house of justice"). These aspirations became enshrined in the 1906/11 Constitution, but it was after the accession of Reza Shah Pahlavi to the throne in 1925 that a modern Iranian judiciary was established that included written laws, court proceedings, and trained western-style judges and legal professionals. Since the French system was used as a model, the body of pre-1979 laws combined concepts from the 1804 French Civil Code. Islamic law was applicable to inheritance and family matters.[46] Most importantly, a new criminal law replaced the Shariʿa and in later years, elements of family law were also reformed and modernized, such as giving women the right to divorce and custody. After the revolution, the earlier reformed family and criminal laws were considered un-Islamic and changed to comply with the tenets of Shariʿa. As Article 4 of the post-1979 Constitution stipulates, all Iranian laws must be based on "Islamic criteria, with Shariʿa as its primary source." By and large, the civil domains of the law remain as in pre-revolutionary era.

Article 156 of the current Constitution stipulates the independence of the judiciary from other branches of the government. Yet, the Supreme Leader appoints the Head of the Judiciary, who then appoints the heads of the provincial courts, who in turn appoint lower-ranking judges. Hence, all judges effectively owe their allegiance to the Supreme Leader. "Only clerics who trained in Islamic jurisprudence, or have degrees from religious law schools, can become judges.[47] Women are barred from becoming judges altogether. The head of the judiciary, the country's prosecutor general, and all Supreme Court judges have to be *mojtahids*, or high-ranking clerics."

The *Majlis* passes laws, provided these are approved by the

---

[46] R. Banakar and K. Ziaee, "The Life of the Law in the Islamic Republic of Iran", *Iranian Studies*, vol. 51, no. 5, 26 June 2018, pp. 717-746, DOI: 10.1080/00210862.2018.1467266.

[47] H. Ghaemi, "The Islamic Judiciary", *The Iran Primer*, 6 October 2010.

Guardian Council, which ensures that the laws conform with the Shari'a. Customs and usages (*'urf*) play a limited role and only then when a codified law is not available. "Thus, the Iranian legal system is a hybrid of Shari'a on the one hand, and civil law institutions and procedures on the other." Though the spirit of due process is enshrined in the Constitution, "the principle of the rule of law (*hākemiyyat-e qānun*) is "largely absent from Iranian constitutional doctrine. Instead, the rule of Shari'a and the principle of *velāyat-e faqih* play decisive roles in shaping the boundaries of law and legality."[48]

The World Justice Project and Rule of Law Index

To evaluate objectively how strong or weak the Iranian legal environment actually is, it is important to benchmark it against other countries. To this end, this article relies on the World Justice Project (WJP) Rule of Law Index, which in its 2020 report covers 128 countries and jurisdictions, and thus serves as a quantitative tool for measuring the rule of law in practice.[49]

"Rule of law" is difficult to define and to measure. It can differ from one society or culture to another. For the purposes of producing a quantitative and qualitative index, WJP convened practitioners from seventeen professional disciplines (judges, lawyers, police, etc.), academics, and community leaders from more than one hundred countries. These experts, all directly involved in the practice of law, agreed on a common definition, and vetted the methodology for the index. The focus of the index is the adherence to the rule of law from the perspective of ordinary individuals and their experiences with a host of everyday situations in their societies.

The data for the index are derived for each report in two ways: (1) a General Population Poll conducted by leading local polling companies, using a representative sample of over 1,000

---

[48] R. Banakar and K. Ziae (2018).
[49] World Justice Project, "World Justice Project Rule of Law Index 2020", 2020.

respondents, roughly equal numbers of men and women, in the three largest cities of each country; and (2) a technical questionnaire completed by in-country legal practitioners and experts. The 2020 index is based on over 130,000 household surveys and 4,000 practitioner responses, globally. Undoubtedly, it is the most comprehensive dataset of its kind and covers 44 areas of the law organized under the following eight headings, which are scored and ranked:

1. Constraints on Government Powers,
2. Absence of Corruption,
3. Open Government,
4. Fundamental Rights,
5. Order and Security,
6. Regulatory Enforcement,
7. Civil Justice, and
8. Criminal Justice.

The dimensions examined reveal whether the laws are "clear, publicized, and stable; are applied evenly; and protect fundamental rights, including the security of persons and contract, property, and human rights. Whether the processes by which the laws are enacted, administered, and enforced are accessible, fair, and efficient. Whether justice is delivered timely by competent, ethical, and independent representatives and neutrals who are accessible, have adequate resources, and reflect the makeup of the communities they serve".

Iran's Standing

No society is flawless. Strengthening the rule of law is a major responsibility of governments. It requires a continuous effort to build, maintain, correct, and update institutions, capacities, and standards that promote a culture for respect of the rule of law. The Netherlands and the four Scandinavian countries come on top of the 2020 WJP rankings; the United States ranks 21st.

Data from Iran were obtained from respondents in Tehran, Mashhad, and Isfahan – the three largest cities. Iran's overall ranking is 109 out of the 128 comparators in the 2020 report. It ranks low in general, and particularly so when compared to its regional and global peers: it is 7th out of the eight MENA countries in the report, and 41st among the 42 in the middle-income category, to which Iran belongs. Its worst score relates to fundamental rights, and within this category[50] freedom of religion (0.05) right to privacy (0.12), and freedom of associations (0.12) score among the lowest in the world. [51] Iran's highest score is in order and security, which is lifted by the score of absence of civil conflict (0.85) and absence of crime (0.76). Respondents scored the experience with civil law, which is based largely on the pre-revolutionary codes, higher than criminal justice, which was revamped to comply with Shari'a. Unsurprisingly, the score for corruption is high; particularly the corruption score in the judiciary (.54) and in the police/military (.52).

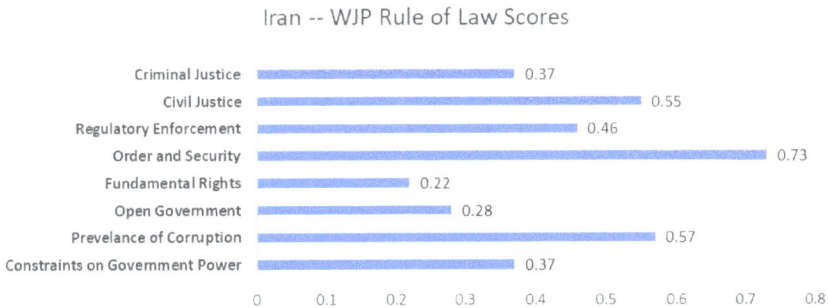

Iran -- WJP Rule of Law Scores

Criminal Justice	0.37
Civil Justice	0.55
Regulatory Enforcement	0.46
Order and Security	0.73
Fundamental Rights	0.22
Open Government	0.28
Prevelance of Corruption	0.57
Constraints on Government Power	0.37

Source: World Justice Report, 2020[52]

---

[50] Ibid., p. 89.

[51] Ibid.

[52] Ibid.

Conclusion

Plagues and pandemics have changed the course of history around the world and caused social, economic, and political transformations. The Black Plague in Europe eroded the power of the Catholic Church and led to the Reformation, ended the institution of serfdom, and ushered in the age of the enlightenment.

Today, COVID19 has exposed every country's dysfunctions, vulnerabilities, and fault lines. In the political realm, governments will be judged by their constituents on how they responded to the pandemic. Just as the over 250,000 Covid-19 deaths in the United States reduced the odds of President Trump's re-election, so too will the heavy loss of lives and livelihoods play a role in Iran's 2021 presidential election and the legitimacy of the regime.

The dissatisfaction with the regime is running high on many fronts. The economy is doing poorly, poverty and income inequality is rising, unemployment rate is climbing. Meanwhile the frequent mega-corruption by regime insiders and their circles of family and friends, the misogyny, the infringement on personal freedoms, the differential access to justice, and the regime's heavy-handedness toward any expression of discontent are among the causes that widen the identity gap between the citizens and their aging leadership.

While advanced and emerging countries have struggled with the impact of COVID19, it has been disproportionately high on Iranians. As bilateral and multilateral agencies joined forces to support affected countries in every way possible, Iran was not only left to face the pandemic on its own but to do so with its hands tied behind its back because of America's 'maximum pressure' sanctions, which are tied to the regional policies of the regime. There have been numerous reports about shortages of critical medications (e.g. insulin) or necessary inputs for domestic pharma producers, even though these items were presumably exempted from the sanctions.

Despite backbreaking constraints and the heavy sacrifices average Iranians have made, religious authorities have downplayed the impact, countered public health efforts, and attacked vigorously any criticism. For instance, just recently, in the city of Mashhad, a disabled body builder was arrested and threatened with execution when he questioned the inconsistencies in Covid restrictions which allowed shrines to stay open and ordered gyms to close.[53]

The writing on the wall is clear that no country will return to its pre-pandemic normal and Covid-19 will accelerate the pace for change and transformation. Iran will not be an exception and Iranians want change in every aspect. Whether this change will be facilitated in a peaceful or conflictual way will shape the trajectory of the country as it begins a new century according to the Persian calendar. The next six to nine months will be a turning point.

In the English town of Weymouth is a plaque stating that the Black Plague entered England through this port in 1348. It killed nearly half of the country's population and resulted in the people losing faith in the Church as an ineffectual institution already mired in corruption. History will note that the 2020 Covid-19 pandemic entered Iran through Qom.

---

[53] "Iran arrests disabled bodybuilder over criticism of coronavirus rules: report", *i24News*, 10 November 2020.

Conclusions

Karim Mezran and Annalisa Perteghella

While reporting fewer cases than other, harder-hit, regions such as Europe, the Middle East and North Africa region is likely to be equally impacted by the long-term consequences of the pandemic.

The reason for the relatively low number of cases reported has been attributed alternatively to a warmer climate (even though there is no scientific proof of a correlation between outside temperature and the possibility of contracting the virus) and a significantly younger population, which presents less symptoms and less long-term consequences than older people who instead make up most of the European population. Another reason for the low numbers is believed to be underreporting, whether intentional or due to a lack of preparedness and ability to test.

Among the countries analyzed in this Report, Iran is without doubt the one that is paying the highest price, with about 600,000 reported cases and more than 30,000 deaths at the end of October. Iraq too is reporting one of the highest number of cases in the region (500,000, with 10,000 deaths), which is likely due to its geographical proximity to and high number of daily exchanges with Iran. As for North African countries, Egypt reported about 107,000 cases with 2,000 deaths, while Libya and Algeria declared very similar numbers (60,000 cases with 1,000 deaths for Libya and 2,000 deaths for Algeria). In the GCC, Saudi Arabia is the country most affected, with 346,000 reported cases and more than 5,000 deaths, followed by Qatar (132,000 cases and 230 deaths), the UAE (130,000 cases and 500 deaths), Kuwait (123,000 cases and 800 deaths), Oman (115,000 cases and 1,200 deaths), and Bahrain (81,000 cases and 317 deaths).

Despite apparently being less hard-hit, the actual impact and consequences of the pandemic on states in the MENA region are set to be huge. Of course, it is not possible to make generalizations for the whole region, which remains as heterogenous as ever: MENA countries differ in terms of GDP and health infrastructures, and some of them suffer from political instability and sometimes violent conflicts.

Exactly as with humans, which are hit hardest when presenting pre-existing conditions, MENA states have been impacted because of their pre-existing conditions. In this sense, the Covid-19 pandemic has laid bare all the vulnerabilities and deficiencies of these states' structures, and has aggravated pre-existing political, social, and economic shortcomings.

While the impact, and the possible consequences, of the pandemic are different for each state, some common features can be highlighted:

- By failing to provide an adequate response to the pandemic, states' authorities are experiencing a further loss in legitimacy, which adds to the pre-existing contestation and risks of giving rise to a further wave of protests.

- In many regional states, protests were already underway and have only been stopped by the pandemic and the government-imposed curfews and social distancing measures. Despite a short-term gain in time for governments, they are much likely to explode again once the virus has been contained, this time fueled by the grievances highlighted above and by the precipitating economic crisis.

- Many governments in the region have been using the emergency powers granted by the need to manage the pandemic to further crack down on domestic opposition and strengthen anti-terrorism laws, ultimately curbing fundamental freedoms. Again, while these measures give an advantage to political regimes in the short term, they are likely to be met with further discontent over the medium term.

- As elsewhere, the pandemic has strengthened and increased the role of the state, but in the MENA region it happens at a time in which the state is under growing pressure both from its citizens and by non-state actors, exactly for its lack of ability to manage ordinary life.

- Partial exemption to these dynamics are the GCC states, where there is no organized, grassroots opposition to ruling governments, and where the huge financial resources these states have access to could help in softening the economic impact of the pandemic over the short term. However, for GCC states, too, the crisis looms on the horizon, as the double shock due to the collapse of oil prices and Covid-19 has renewed the urgency of achieving economic diversification and, with it, a reform of the social compact, transitioning away from the Arab authoritarian compact based on the principle of "no taxation without representation."

There is a lively debate going on about whether the pandemic is a geopolitical game-changer or a mere accelerator of dynamics that were already underway. For the MENA region, we can say that for the moment it is significantly revealing all the cracks in the states' structures, and over the next months this could translate into an acceleration of those dynamics of protest and contestation that were already rife before the pandemic started.

Ten years after the Arab Spring, a second wave of uprisings, which took off in 2019 and has only temporarily been halted by the pandemic, is about to regain full steam. Protests in Algeria and Iraq have already resumed. In Egypt, too, rare protests against the government have been launched, despite the harsh wave of arrests sparked by the 2019 protests. Libya has been witnessing widespread and nationwide protests since August. In the Persian Gulf region, for the moment there is no report of mass protests, but smoldering discontent can soon reignite another wave of demonstrations in Iran, while in the GCC countries discontent will probably continue to be voiced online.

As the pandemic-induced crisis is expected to exacerbate poverty and inequalities, the poor response by state authorities and the strengthening of authoritarian practices is most likely to amplify dynamics and reasons for discontent, thus transforming the coronavirus crisis from a health crisis into an economic and political one.

About the Authors

Emadeddin Badi is a nonresident senior fellow with the Middle East Program at the Atlantic Council, where he focuses primarily on U.S and European policies towards Libya and the wider geopolitical implications of the conflict. Previously, he was a nonresident scholar at the Counterterrorism and Extremism Program at the Middle East Institute. Badi is an independent consultant who has worked with multiple development and international organizations as well as private sector stakeholders with a focus on Libya. From 2015 to 2018, he gained hands-on experience programming the conflict-sensitive implementation of a flagship stabilization initiative implemented across Libya for UNDP. Mr. Badi has also worked on multiple research and policy-oriented projects with various institutions, with an extensive focus on Libya's non-state actors. Most recently, he co-authored a paper on the *Development of Libya's Armed Groups Since 2014 – Community Dynamics and Economic Interests with the Royal Institute of International Affairs* – Chatham House. He is also currently affiliated with the School of Transnational Governance at the European University Institute in Florence, Italy, where he focuses on EU policy towards Libya.

Gawdat Bahgat is professor of National Security Affairs at the National Defense University's Near East South Asia Center for Strategic Study. He is an Egyptian-born specialist in Middle Eastern policy, particularly Egypt, Iran, and the Gulf region. His areas of expertise include energy security, proliferation of weapons of mass destruction, counter-terrorism, Arab-Israeli conflict, North Africa, and American foreign policy in the Middle East. Before joining NESA in December 2009, he taught at different universities. Bahgat published eight books including *Energy Security* (2011), *International Political Economy* (2010), *Proliferation of Nuclear Weapons in the Middle East* (2007), *Israel and the Persian Gulf* (2006), and *American Oil Diplomacy* (2003). His work has been translated to several foreign languages. Bahgat served as an advisor to several governments and oil companies.

Nadereh Chamlou is a retired Senior Advisor to the Chief Economist at the World Bank's Middle East and North Africa Region. During her over three decade career, she worked in technical, advisory, coordination, and managerial positions across the World Bank Group in areas such as economic management, private and financial sector development, infrastructure, corporate governance, and gender. Mrs. Chamlou has regional expertise particularly in Middle East and North Africa, but her regional experience also extends to Latin America, East Asia, the Pacific, and Eastern Europe. She co-authored a World Bank flagship report titled *Corporate Governance: A Framework for Implementation* (1999) and co-founded the World Bank/OECD sponsored Global Corporate Governance Forum which she headed its Secretariat from 1998-2000. In 2013, she authored a working paper titled, *Iran's Unrealised Potential – Its Underutilised Talent Pool.* Today, she works as an International Development Advisor in Washington, DC.

Hafsa Halawa is a nonresident scholar at the Middle East Institute and an independent consultant working on political, social and economic affairs, and development goals across the MENA, and Horn of Africa regions. A former corporate lawyer, Halawa has held positions in government, the UN, INGOs/NGOs, corporate multinationals, private firms, and think tanks. She now consults independently for a similar broad set of clients on a variety of issues, at request. She holds an LLB from the University of Exeter and an LLM from University College London/Queen Mary's University.

Abbas Kadhim leads the Atlantic Council's Iraq Initiative. He is an Iraq expert and author of *Reclaiming Iraq: The 1920 Revolution and the Founding of the Modern State*. Most recently, he was a senior foreign policy fellow at Johns Hopkins University's School of Advanced International Studies. He was formerly an assistant professor of national security affairs and Middle East studies at the Naval Postgraduate School in Monterey, California and a visiting assistant professor at Stanford University. He also previously held a senior government affairs position at the Iraqi Embassy in Washington, DC. His books include Governance in the Middle East and North Africa and The Hawza Under Siege: Studies in the Ba'th Party Archive. He earned a PhD in Near Eastern Studies from the University of California, Berkeley.

Yahia Mohamed Lamine Mestek, PhD, is associate professor at DBKM University, and head of the Department of Political Science, where he is responsible for post-graduate and scientific research. He is also a Member of the International Consortium for Geopolitical Studies of the Sahel (ICGPS) and a Leaders for Democracy fellow at Maxwell School of Citizenship and Public Affairs at Syracuse University. Mr. Mestek is the author of scholarly articles on Algerian politics and regional affairs in the Mediterranean, including "Algerian Foreign Policy Facing Upheavals in the Mediterranean Region" published in the Algerian journal Voice of the Law. He pursued a PhD in Political Sciences and International Relation from Algiers 3 University.

Karim Mezran is a resident senior fellow with the Atlantic Council's Rafik Hariri Center for the Middle East. As a distinguished Libyan-Italian scholar, he brings significant depth of understanding to the processes of political change in North Africa. He is also an adjunct professor of Middle East Studies at the Johns Hopkins University School of Advanced International Studies (SAIS). Previously, he was director of the Center for American Studies in Rome. His analyses on the Middle East and North Africa have been widely published in Italian- and other-language journals and publications. Mr. Mezran holds a PhD in international relations from SAIS.

Annalisa Perteghella, PhD, is a research fellow for the Middle East and North Africa Centre at ISPI. She is an expert on Middle Eastern politics, and on Europe-Middle East relations. Her recent work focuses on international security, political violence, conflict analysis, and prevention, as well as the role of foresight and evaluation in European foreign policy. She is also the Scientific Coordinator of the Rome MED Dialogues, the high-level project on the wider Mediterranean region co-promoted by ISPI and the Italian Ministry of Foreign Affairs and International Cooperation, bringing together heads of state, ministers, international organizations as well as high-level representatives from the private sector, academia, think tanks, and civil society. She obtained her PhD in Politics and Institutions from the Catholic University in Milan. Her doctoral research focused on the study of religious and political authority in Iran since the 1979 revolution. She is the author and editor of articles and chapters in books, among the most recent: *Russia's Relations with Iran, Saudi Arabia and Turkey: Friends in Need, Friends Indeed?*, in C. Lovotti, E. Tafuro Ambrosetti, C. Hartwell, A. Chmielewska (Eds); *Russia in the Middle East and North Africa. Continuity and Change* (2020); *Iran: An Unrecognized Regional Power*, in S. Giusti and I. Mirkina (Eds); and *The EU in a Trans-European Space* (2019).